TRAGIC FAILURES

The Romanell Lectures

The Romanell–Phi Beta Kappa Professorship, first awarded in 1983, was established by an endowment from Patrick and Edna Romanell. Patrick Romanell, a Phi Beta Kappa member from Brooklyn College, was H. Y. Benedict Professor of Philosophy at the University of Texas, El Paso. The Phi Beta Kappa Society administers the professorship, which takes the form of three lectures given each year by a distinguished philosopher, at his or her home institution, on a topic important to an audience beyond professional philosophers. This intent of this series is to publish the results of those lectures in affordable and accessible editions.

Tragic Failures
How and Why We are Harmed by Toxic Chemicals
Carl F. Cranor

What do Philosophers Do?
Skepticism and the Practice of Philosophy
Penelope Maddy

TRAGIC FAILURES

How and Why We are Harmed
by Toxic Chemicals

Carl F. Cranor

OXFORD
UNIVERSITY PRESS

OXFORD
UNIVERSITY PRESS

Oxford University Press is a department of the University of Oxford. It furthers
the University's objective of excellence in research, scholarship, and education
by publishing worldwide. Oxford is a registered trade mark of Oxford University
Press in the UK and certain other countries.

Published in the United States of America by Oxford University Press
198 Madison Avenue, New York, NY 10016, United States of America.

© Oxford University Press 2017

Library of Congress Cataloging-in-Publication Data
Names: Cranor, Carl F., author.
Title: Tragic failures: how and why we are harmed by toxic
chemicals / Carl F. Cranor.
Description: New York, NY: Oxford University Press, [2017]
Identifiers: LCCN 2016042228 | ISBN 9780190635756 (hardcover) |
ISBN 9780190635770 (epub)
Subjects: LCSH: Toxicological chemistry—United States. |
Environmental health—United States. | Public health—Political aspects—
United States. | Health risk assessment—United States.
Classification: LCC RA1219.3 .C73 2017 | DDC 616.9—dc23
LC record available at https://lccn.loc.gov/2016042228

CONTENTS

PREFACE

Perhaps too often we are surprised when members of the public noticeably suffer diseases or dysfunctions from exposures to toxic substances. They rarely seem to make the news but are concerning when they do. However, toxic substances likely cause many more diseases than are publicly conveyed, and they surely cause more than are reported as subject to action by public health agencies or as legal actions in the tort law.

On the public health side, laws that are supposed to protect citizens from toxicity-caused diseases accomplish this so poorly that we rarely read of the US Environmental Protection Agency, the Occupational Safety and Health administration, or the Consumer Product Safety Commission taking action to better protect us. There are several reasons for this. In the 1970s Congress created laws that hamper this effort; the 1976 Toxic Substances Control Act (TSCA) deserves special mention because of its shortcomings. Another is that the science needed to justify legal action can be difficult to produce even under the best circumstances but is exacerbated in the current legal environment. A third reason is that the laws create ignorance about potential toxicants, provide substantial incentives for companies to remain ignorant about their own products, and, because of the legal structures, provide many incentives for companies to create doubt about the science or demand ideal science in fiercely opposing any actions that might threaten their products or reduce their profits.

When people are actually harmed by toxicants, the tort or personal injury law can face somewhat similar problems. This area of the law has developed over time for the purpose of redressing harms one citizen causes to another (or others). Yet, despite popular myths that people sue too much and that it is easy to win judgments against companies, neither is true. This is particularly the case once one understands some changes in the tort law, how it is administered, the science needed for tort law redress, and some of the difficulties that injured parties face in succeeding with their litigation.

There are some similarities between problems in the two areas of the law that hinder public health protections in the first place and then frustrate redress in the tort law when preventive efforts fail. Since my research has focused on how science is utilized in the two areas of the law, it seemed that that common themes should be developed and extended in a more publicly accessible book in order to explain some of the main, but hidden, issues that importantly affect our health.

The National Phi Beta Kappa Society provided this opportunity with my selection as the Romanell–Phi Beta Kappa Professor in Philosophy for 2014–2015.[1] Part of this award consisted of giving three special lectures of one's choice at one's home institution. This I did at the University of California, Riverside (UCR), under the aegis of the Iota Chapter of Phi Beta Kappa of California and the UCR Honors Program. These lectures were given beginning in October 2014, under a different title. The lectures grew out of, reflect, and develop further research I have conducted on philosophic issues at the interface of science, law, and philosophy for more than 30 years. While this has been my research area, it is also one in which I have participated in various public venues—on science advisory panels, in legal conferences, before regulatory agencies, and in some courts of law. Although it might not be apparent on its face how science is utilized in a variety of legal forums, institutional choices about when and how science should be used can have major consequences for citizens. This book describes some of these consequences. I hope that this work provides some illumination for ideas about the use of science in two important areas of the law that can so profoundly affect our lives and health.

As this book was in the final stages of publication Congress, otherwise known for its gridlock and opposition to regulatory protections for the public, surprisingly amended the 1976 TSCA with the Frank R. Lautenberg Chemical Safety for the 21st Century Act.[2] The Lautenberg Act created a premarket toxicity testing law with improved deadlines for reviewing existing products that many, including the author, had long advocated. Consequently, in order to respond to the legal changes, I had to modify the arc of argument in various places. Prior to the Lautenberg Act, the 1976 TSCA (and other laws) failed to protect the public's health well from toxicants.

In order to understand some of the complex legal and scientific issues during this transition period we should recognize the legal shortcomings in the 1976 TSCA (and I did not change that). Chapters 1 and 2 focus on shortcomings of earlier legislation that permitted substantial risks to the public health. In Chapter 4, I review improvements and likely consequences of the new Lautenberg Act going forward. It requires that the EPA make an affirmative finding that new products do not pose unreasonable risks to the public. Thus, new chemicals should be much safer from 2017 onward as they receive legitimate premarket reviews. However, modifications for addressing substances already in commerce must be implemented against the background of forty years of considerable ignorance about chemical creations that developed during this time. Providing better safeguards for the public, despite amendments that provide more aggressive reviews of products and legally enforceable time lines to remove toxic risks, will be an enormous task that likely will take a very long time. The 1976 TSCA has created a chemical soup of known and unknown toxicity that must be addressed by the postmarket, postexposure provisions of the Lautenberg Act. Will it be able to overcome problems that developed under the previous version of TSCA?

Acknowledgements: A number of people made possible the Romanell–Phi Beta Kappa Professorship and Lectures, for which I am grateful. My philosophy and Phi Beta Kappa colleague, John Martin Fischer, nominated me on behalf of the chapter for this award, and I very much appreciate his support. Gladys Herrera-Berkowitz provided support for the application and stayed in contact with Phi Beta Kappa. Myra Jones assisted with the logistics of the lectures. Rich Cardullo, director of the Honors Program, wonderfully provided institutional support and ideas for the lectures. Thanks to him the presentation on the tort law was given at a court where litigation occurs, at a century-old courtroom in Riverside's historic courthouse. It was a delight to work with John Churchill, the national secretary of Phi Beta Kappa, and to be introduced by him at the courthouse lecture.

I am quite grateful to two academic colleagues who have supported and helped inform my research over many years. I learned much from David A. Eastmond of the Environmental Toxicology Graduate Program. When I had the beginnings of an idea about toxicology and how it might function in the law, he often confirmed it, other times modified it and made it more precise, and sometimes steered me away from a misleading one. My philosophy colleague Larry Wright has been similarly valuable because of his abiding interest in and work on inferences to the best explanation, about which we have had many conversations. This standard form of inference sometimes seems mysterious or we may not fully understand how it works, yet it is central to scientific and many other inferences, but tort law judges have not always allowed its use in their courtroom. Thanks to conversations with and work by Larry, my research and some testimony in legal cases has helped make the law more receptive to this centuries-old inference that we all use. Finally, my thanks to David A. Eastmond, Heinrik Hellwig, Taylor J. Cranor, and Crystal A. Cranor for reading aspects of the manuscript in preparation. All provided invaluable comments that found their way into the book. Over many years of research I have also learned much from colleagues who are legal scholars, scientists, public health officials, philosophers, and practicing lawyers too numerous to mention, but I wish to generically express my gratitude for their friendship and contributions. Peter Ohlin, philosophy editor at Oxford University Press, merits substantial thanks for being very supportive of this project and helpful at critical points as it was being completed.

Introduction

In 1998 Jeromy Darling, then 26, was riding his bicycle inside his workplace, a large DuPont plant in Parkersburg, West Virginia, when he accidentally fell on its crossbar and hit his groin. While short-term pain from such an event is not unusual, his did not disappear. Consulting a doctor, he was diagnosed with testicular cancer, and he had to have one testicle removed along with a number of "lymph nodes from his abdomen."[1] The operation cost him $75,000, leading to bankruptcy as a consequence.

Darling's co-worker Ken Wamsley, "a lab analyst in the Teflon division" also suffered health problems. The chemical from which Teflon and hundreds of other products were made, known as C8 or perfluorooctanoic acid (PFOA), "' . . . was everywhere,' . . . bubbling out of the glass flasks he used to transport it, wafting into a smelly vapor that formed when he heated it. A fine powder, possibly C8, dusted the laboratory drawers and floated in the hazy lab air."[2] At the time neither he nor other coworkers thought much about the vapor or the fine powder in their workplace.[3] He believed it was harmless, " . . . like a soap. Wash your hands [with it], your face, take a bath."[4] "Today Wamsley suffers from ulcerative colitis, a bowel condition that causes him sudden bouts of diarrhea. The disease also can—and in his case, did—lead to rectal cancer. Between surgery in 2002, which left him reliant on plastic pouches that collect his waste outside his body and have to be changed regularly, and his ongoing digestive problems, Wamsley finds it difficult to be away from his home for long."[5] Later he had doubts about C8's safety and "his bosses' casual assurances.... 'When did they know? Did they lie?' "[6] Ulcerative colitis is a known disease from C8 exposure.[7]

In 1999 a local Parkersburg rancher, Wilbur Tennant, contacted a lawyer because a stream running from property he had sold to DuPont for a "non-hazardous landfill" turned "smelly and black with a layer of foam floating on the surface."[8] Tennant's cattle drank from the stream, which contained concentrations of C8 100 times greater than DuPont's own internal standards regarded as safe. Within a short time, "hundreds of [his] cattle had died."[9] DuPont's internal studies had shown that C8 was quite capable of killing or sickening experimental animals at various concentrations.

Carla Bartlett of nearby Guysville, Ohio, drank tap water contaminated with C8. Later she developed kidney cancer. In the first tort law or personal injury case to go to trial for C8 exposures, a jury awarded her 1.6 million dollars.[10]

While Darling, Wamsley, Bartlett, and Tennant's cattle have little else in common, they all were exposed to C8. All of them contracted diseases that are now clearly linked to the C8 exposures.

How do we know this? Numerous internal memos and other information found during discovery in the tort suit revealed that DuPont knew from internal testing that C8 was toxic (1961), that it accumulated in employees' bodies and elevated liver enzymes (1978), and that it had been "pooped," as one of DuPont's lawyers put it, into "the river and into drinking water," and had also contaminated the air.[11] DuPont settled the suit on behalf of about 80,000 area residents that could eventually amount to about $343 million.[12]

The tort settlement also established an independent scientific panel to oversee studies between C8 exposure and a limited number of diseases. C8 is "associated with kidney and testicular cancer,"[13] ulcerative colitis, high cholesterol, pregnancy-induced hypertension, and thyroid disease.[14] Apparently, numerous other diseases, outside the settlement agreement, have been linked to C8—"ovarian cancer; prostate cancer; lymphoma; reduced fertility; arthritis; hyperactivity and altered immune responses in children; and hypotonia, or 'floppiness,' in infants."[15]

More broadly, 99.7% of the rest of us have detectable concentrations of C8 in our bodies. Not all of us will necessarily be at risk, but this datum is powerful evidence of C8's ubiquitous presence. Moreover, it has spread all over the world, from polar bears to pandas to people, and from the central Pacific Ocean to coastal waters.[16]

THE LAW

Why were these people and cattle harmed? Aren't chemical products tested for their safety before employees, the public, or cattle are exposed? After all, we take prescription drugs with considerable confidence that they will relieve or cure our afflictions without undue risks. If we use some of the myriad products containing C8—nonstick cookware, stain-resistant fabrics and upholstery, and Gore-Tex, to name a few—and if employees work with the raw chemicals, surely they must be legally tested for their toxicity before there are exposures? The short answer is, "No."

Because we know pharmaceuticals are tested for their beneficial and potentially toxic side effects, we might have the same trust in the chemical components of hair products, cosmetics, water bottles, nonstick frying pans, couches, baby bottles, car seats, building materials, and the safety of our workplaces. We might, but we shouldn't.

What's the difference between prescription drugs and those other everyday chemicals? In two words: the law. In a few more words: the law creates and invites ignorance about toxicants, risking our health and permitting substantial harm.

For prescription drugs, Congress created laws that require tests for their safety and effectiveness *prior to* entering the market. Thus, scientists and health officials understand the main properties of the approved chemicals, their benefits, and their possible risks.

In contrast, the major 1976 public health law governing general chemical products—the Toxic Substances Control Act (TSCA)—forbade blanket *premarket* toxicity testing and review of more than 22,000 new chemical products that have subsequently entered the market. It also grandfathered as "safe" 62,000 existing substances, including C8. The list of 62,000 includes chemicals manufactured or imported into the United States, excluding comparatively small numbers of prescription drugs, pesticides, tobacco products, nuclear material, foods, new food additives, chemical mixtures, and cosmetic ingredients. We are largely ignorant about these creations, their properties, and the risks they pose. Knowing this, do you still have confidence in the safety of such products in your home or your workplace?

The law is not the only institution that contributes to such risks. Laws provide the rules of the game for protecting the public, or, one might say, prescribe the relations between people in the community. But science also plays an important role in discovering, understanding, limiting, and mitigating risks. It offers important empirical evidence in different legal venues to help assess whether or not the laws have been carried out and how well they protect us. Laws differ in specifying *when* and *how much* science should be used to protect the public. If chemical products pose risks or cause harm, how science is used in the law and how it is administered can either put us at risk or better protect us. Citizens can be treated justly or unjustly as a result.

In another area of the law—the tort or personal-injury law—if individuals have actually been harmed, as Carla Bartlett was, similar relationships between the law and science and judicial decisions implementing them substantially affect our lives. The administration of science in the tort law could too easily thwart redress of injuries, or, conversely, better facilitate just compensation for wrongful harm. Which one occurs depends on what science the law requires and how courts choose to administer it.

To sharpen these issues, consider some other examples.

FORMALDEHYDE

Citizens are exposed daily to formaldehyde, a known human carcinogen, and have been for decades.[17] Formaldehyde is present in many consumer products—home and trailer house construction, haircare products, insulation, wallpaper, paints, fabrics, draperies, wooden-floor finishes, and laminated flooring.[18] Some people living in house trailers constructed of plywood, which uses formaldehyde in a wood adhesive, after Hurricane Katrina destroyed their own homes, experienced "burning eyes, sore throats and other more serious ailments."[19] Similarly, in 2015 laminated flooring sold by Lumber Liquidators emitted high levels of formaldehyde exceeding California's standards, according to a CBS 60 Minutes report. "[L]ong-term exposure at that level would be risky because it would increase the risk for chronic respiratory irritation, change a person's lung function, [and] increase [the] risk of asthma. It's not going to produce symptoms in everyone but children will be the people most likely to show symptoms at that sort of level,"[20] according to Dr. Philip J. Landrigan of the Mt. Sinai Medical Center.

Products for hair smoothing and straightening have contained high concentrations of formaldehyde, and stylists using them experienced nosebleeds and respiratory problems. Sandy Guest, a hairdresser who used Brazilian Blowout, which was "loaded with formaldehyde," became sick and eventually died of leukemia, a known outcome of exposure.[21] Employees at the manufacturing plants would have been at greater risk.

Haircare products receive even less regulatory attention than other substances. These are part of generic "cosmetics" and include lipsticks, eye and facial makeup, cleansing shampoos, permanent waves, and deordants that have intimate contact with our bodies. There is no premarket approval of them. Companies need not inform the Food and Drug Administratin of their ingredients (even formaldehyde in hair products?). They must ensure the safety of their own products and voluntarily choose to withdraw any risky ones. The FDA may not recall particular products. The company fox is in charge of the chicken house and decides when the chickens might be harmed, but it was not soon enough for Sandy Guest. Eventually formaldehyde was removed from Brazilian Blowout.

What has been done to reduce risks from formaldehyde?

In 1981 the US National Toxicology Program (NTP), the main US agency that identifies substances that are toxic, classified formaldehyde as a likely human carcinogen. Thirty years later it upgraded its assessment: formaldehyde is a "known human carcinogen."[22] Between those dates more than 17 studies revealed that people were contracting cancers "of the nasopharyngeal region, sinonasal cavities, and myeloid leukemia."[23] Studies in animal experiments reinforced those findings.

From this research scientists concluded that formaldehyde is quite toxic to human beings. Their findings informed a community of experts. Public health officials surely knew of formaldehyde's carcinogenicity. Yet, no public, nationwide legal standards or restrictions on its use have been set (see chapter 1).

Could the US Environmental Protection Agency (EPA) have implemented public health protections within a decade or less after formaldehyde was judged a probable human carcinogen? This seems plausible. Yet public health protections languish. Formaldehyde has been under review by the EPA's risk group, the Integrated Risk Information System (IRIS), on and off and on for 35 years.[24] Why? Our current laws led to this outcome. They permit products of unknown toxicity to be sold to the public, leaving people exposed to any that turn out to be toxic until a health agency not only has sufficient evidence of toxicity but also manages to overcome regulatory obstruction and to issue improved health protections. Fortunately, California homeowners who had installed Lumber Liquidator's laminated flooring had some legal protections from the state that homeowners from other areas of the country did not.[25]

The law also tempts companies to do all they can to hinder protections and even confound the science. Companies demand the very best and most certain, even ideal, scientific evidence, which has the result of postponing legal action (chapter 4). They also pay "white-coat scientists" for hire to assist them. They often call on politicians to slow assessments simply to protect their products; sometimes they manipulate or falsify data (chapter 1).[26]

ROUNDUP

Other countries have developed more effective means of protecting the public from toxic exposures. In March 2015, the World Health Organization's International Agency for Research on Cancer (IARC) classified the pesticide Roundup (technical name "glyphosate"; made by the international conglomerate Monsanto) as a probable carcinogen, the same assessment formaldehyde received in 1981. Within three months the French minister of ecology, in a country with different laws than the United States, banned it from sale in self-service aisles in garden shops and nurseries.[27] Thus, France provided partial protection from Roundup with the legal equivalent of lightning speed. California was able to quickly list Roundup as a carcinogen because of a state warning law that has some important provisions (discussed in chapter 4).

Our laws and powerful political pressures have made for slothful progress on formaldehyde, C8, and many other products. "Slothful" should remain relegated to describing the movements of a manatee, nematode, slug, garden snail, or starfish[28]—it should never characterize the speed at which a government protects its citizens. Such slow protective rates bode ill for the American public.

Existing laws and the way the legal system uses science have produced several undesirable outcomes. There are still no nationwide health standards for C8 in various environmental media, although by now both 3M and DuPont have voluntarily phased it out.[29] While there are some occupational standards for formaldehyde, there are no nationwide, authoritative public health standards.[30] It is listed as a carcinogen and proposed health standards are in process, but there are no clear legal limits.[31] There are some informal guidelines for reducing exposures, advice for buying products, summaries of scientific studies (but no endorsement of their quality), and a few state warnings about exposures.[32] Of course, citizens can review this information and decide what to do, but few products have legal assurances of safety like pharmaceuticals typically do. Are people exposed to toxic amounts of formaldehyde? Are their children at risk? Finally, when the law permits formaldehyde exposure to endanger or sicken people, are they then treated justly?

SCIENCE AND TORT LAW

Sometimes people are not merely put at risk—they are clearly harmed. When this occurs, they can seek redress in the main area of the law for this purpose—personal injury law, or, more formally, the tort law. Unusually, Carla Barnett received quick redress for injures from C8 (more in chapter 3) because of information found during discovery in this case (often the tort law does not function this well).

This was not Brian K. Milward's fate. A refrigerator repairman, he was exposed to life-threatening harm from a known human carcinogen, benzene. In 2004, at the age of 47, he was diagnosed with acute promyelocytic leukemia (APL). This rare variant of acute myelogenous leukemia (AML) annually occurs only once per one million people. While unusual, APL has a comparatively high 12-year survival rate of 70% (other varieties of AML have worse prognoses).

After discovering he had been exposed to benzene in the products of 22 different companies, he and his wife, Linda, filed a tort law suit in the First Federal District Court in Boston, Massachusetts, to redress the injuries they had suffered. They sought compensation for his injuries, medical expenses, and loss of income, along with major life changes and any misery associated with them.

In order to bring this case, they needed a toxicologist who could show that benzene could cause APL. However, in the district court of origin, the judge "excluded" the Milwards' expert from testifying to a jury. Judge George A. O'Toole found that some lines of the scientist's evidence were only "hypotheses"—insufficiently supported by scientific data—and that the toxicologist did not have appropriate human data to support his claim. Testimony based on such evidence was "unreliable," he ruled.[33] The Milwards' attempt at redress for his disease was at an end in this court.

Why did this occur? Partly it resulted from a 1993 change in how legal trials are conducted, and the kinds and amount of science needed for juries to consider expert testimony. Partly it resulted from how the judge understood and administered the rules governing science and testimony in the case.

In a trilogy of US Supreme Court decisions, beginning with *Daubert v. Merrell-Dow Pharmaceuticals* (1993), the Court gave federal judges increased duties to review scientific evidence and expert testimony in litigation, including toxic torts. One aim was to ensure that juries have reliable scientific support to inform their decisions. If there is insufficient evidence on a particular issue, the case does not go to a jury and the plaintiff loses. This was the Milwards' fate.

Their case was not yet at an end, however. They appealed the trial judge's ruling to the First Federal Circuit Court of Appeals, where the Milwards had a different outcome. The appellate court found that the judge had "abused his discretion" in reviewing the science supporting the Milwards' claims.[34] Thus, at the trial court they were treated unjustly (or I will so argue in chapter 3). Importantly, how the judge ruled on the science—on how much and what kind of science the Milwards needed before their experts could testify and the litigation could go to a jury trial—had a decisive role in their legal case and potentially in their lives.

Had the trial court's decision been the final one, it would have raised several important issues. Because the Milwards could not proceed to a jury trial, there could be no judgment that a legal wrong occurred, and there would have been no legally authoritative decision that benzene exposures comparable to his could cause harm. Ignorance about any risks to other employees or to the public from similar products likely would have continued. Finally, because the judge's views and choices about science were mistaken (chapter 3), other courts might also have unwittingly followed his reasoning. The trial court's ruling wrongly denied the Milwards redress, raising an important issue of justice.

JUSTICE

A prominent theory of justice provides us with the resources to assess the justice of two different legal institutions in protecting us from toxicants: public health law and tort law. Justice, with a preeminent role in assessing social and legal institutions, is "the first virtue of social institutions. . . . Each person possesses an inviolability founded on justice that even the welfare of society as a whole cannot override," as John Rawls has argued.[35] According to this theory, I will urge, citizens with sufficient exposure to C8, formaldehyde, benzene, and other harmful substances have been unjustly violated by how the law and science jointly treated them. When laws or institutions are unjust, they "must be reformed,"[36] and I will argue for legal changes in these legal venues in order to make the world safer for its citizens.

THE IMPORTANCE OF HOW SCIENCE IS USED IN THE LAW

The use of science within the law to provide just health protections, both under preventive public health law and compensatory tort law, is central to this book. While ordinarily philosophers think about guns, knives, and blunt objects as some of the bearers of risks and harms, for 30 years I have been concerned about adverse effects from tiny, invisible, undetectable molecular intruders. They can inflict considerable (often quite agonizing) damage, only they are much more difficult to detect than the more visible forms of violence. Diagnosing molecular harms and their causal paths is subtle and complicated. How should we use science in the law to identify and reduce risks from toxic chemical creations to better protect the public? I address aspects of this question in the following chapters.

Although we might not ordinarily think of science and justice together, issues of justice are at stake in *legislative choices* about how law and science should be jointly utilized to prevent diseases, dysfunctions, and death caused by exposures to industrial chemicals. How the law permits decision makers to administer and enforce such laws is also crucial, and how they do so is also important.

Justice is also in the balance in *judges' choices* about what kind and how much science is required in tort cases to support redress for injuries wrongfully caused. We need to understand and then alter how decisions about science are made in both areas.

We should understand how administrative health laws originated and what legislative choices were made for using science. How did the laws create ignorance about toxicants and incentives to obstruct health protections? How well or poorly do they protect the public from chemical creations, some of which, such as C8, formaldehyde, phthalates, benzene, trichloroethylene (TCE), and numerous others, are toxic (chapter 1)?

Early 21st-century scientific understanding of the effects of toxic substances on children makes the amending of public health laws a critically urgent matter. Chemical creations can trigger diseases or dysfunctions in our children at numerous times, from embryonic or fetal or early-life stages through childhood and teenage years, causing afflictions immediately or much later or in future generations (chapter 2). Treating our children justly should be a vital social and legal priority, but it has not been, because of congressional choices about *when* science should be used to protect them. If substances are toxic, postmarket laws provide protections far too late; considerable misery, suffering, and even premature death can occur to affected persons because of legislative choices. Once toxicants are identified, postmarket laws delay better health protections.

Consequently, one major theme of this book is that we need to modify *when* science is used for the public's protection. We should shift from unjust postmarket laws that ineffectively protect the children and adults to those resembling, but not identical to, premarket legislation for pharmaceuticals and pesticides (chapters 2 and 4). It seemed highly unlikely that Congress would amend current laws in the present obstructionist political climate, but as this book is in the final stages of publication Congress has finally done just that: the Frank R. Lautenberg Chemical Safety for the 21st Century Act (the Lautenberg Act) amends the 1976 TSCA, effectively creating a premarket requirement for new chemicals from the date of implementation into the future.[37] This differs somewhat from similar provisions for pharmaceuticals (Chapter 4), but is a major improvement. However, given a 40-year legacy of products of largely unknown toxicity, it will take considerable time for public health agencies to appropriately review existing substances and actually improve chemical safety, despite some amendments to increase the rate of toxicity assessments and health protections. It will be especially important for the EPA to "get the first reviews right" in order to send manufacturers a message that it will strongly enforce the law to protect the public (Chapter 4).

When existing products are toxic and exposures to them must be reduced or removed, public health personnel should not demand or, under lobbying pressure, should not acquiesce in ideal or unrealistic amounts of evidence to carry out this task, although the law may constrain their decisions. Various patterns of evidence short of the ideal can protect the public (chapter 4). Quicker data generation could expedite protections.

Thus, a second major recommendation focuses on *how much* and *what kinds of* evidence are demanded for public health protections. I recommend related approaches for the tort law.

In tort suits, judges, administering the tort law, should make different choices and resist temptations to require injured parties to have ideal or obviously correct science before experts can testify before juries (chapter 3). Both would substantially hamper redress of harm.

In short, I suggest a unified critique both of postmarket public health laws and the tort law. I then propose a somewhat unified science-law solution for both legal venues (chapter 4).

TRAGIC FAILURES

The title of this book invokes the idea of tragic failures. Mere numbers of diseases or premature deaths could numb us to considerable suffering and misery for those sickened by toxicants, such as Darling,

Bartlett, Guest, and Milward. A tragedy is typically an event (or a series of events) that causes substantial and unnecessary suffering or distress—in this case, choices by our leaders in legal institutions and in companies governed by them led to unfortunate outcomes. These institutions are not some immutable part of the universe over which we have no control, but they have been created, designed, and administered by people in the community. We should recognize the role of human decisions in protecting or not protecting our health.

Exposures to man-made chemical creations and pollutants can and do cause serious illnesses and even deaths, as scientists continue to reveal. The examples of C8 exposures underline this. Our children are at even greater risks for diseases than adults. A variety of toxicity-induced diseases are surely tragic to the families involved, as they were to Sandy Guest and her family, and as we will see with Brian Milward (chapter 3). Yet, they are largely invisible because they involve individual families—out of public view, quietly suffering distress, too often not knowing why family members are sick or have died. Yet, they can suffer lifetime burdens and substantial losses that significantly affect their lives.

Typically, those who get sick or die from involuntary exposures to C8, formaldehyde, benzene, phthalates, asbestos, lead, or other substances are random victims of exposures of which they were unaware and ordinarily could do nothing about. (Of course, sometimes, people bring maladies on themselves; for example, through smoking.)

Many toxicity-induced tragedies are the result of choices, either proximate or more remote in time by legislators, judges, scientists, and company officials. Some decision makers could have chosen better to protect the public or made better choices to provide the possibility of redress for injured parties. They have often erred, leading to the suffering of others. Some may have mistakenly but

unwittingly perpetrated harm; others may have knowingly continued the harm, frustrated others rectifying it, or actually brought it
about. And some of them flourished, often quite substantially, by
contributing to fellow citizens' harm. Did they realize the effects of
their decisions? Did they care how they chose? For better protection and just treatment of citizens decision makers must make better choices.

Chapter 1

Industrial Chemicals as Nuisances

*The Rise of Environmental Health Laws
and Their Limitations*

INTRODUCTION

Rivers burst into flames, choking smog shrouded buildings, oil despoiled beaches, and fish died in rivers. These events and others from the 1960s sparked concerns about a deteriorating environment that could also be a source of human harm. Ohio's Cuyahoga River, burning several times between 1950 and 1969, was one poster child of environmental problems; water, ordinarily used to suppress fires, burned. The 1969 spectacle helped motivate legislation to clean up industrial and other wastes in rivers and harbors. The Santa Barbara oil spill sullied the beach and the Pacific Ocean.

Palpable air pollution highlighted public health problems. When I began graduate school at UCLA, smog often burned my eyes and veiled nearby mountains. About 70 miles eastward at my new position at the University of California, noon smog obscured hills not a mile from my office. Runners exercising in smoggy conditions choked on ozone.

Rachel Carson's *Silent Spring*,[38] an early harbinger of environmental problems, which reinforced the above concerns with its warnings, "altered the course of history".[39] While pesticides, and DDT in particular, were prominent in her book, the broader narrative was that invisible toxicants were being released into the environment, harming wildlife and ecosystems, and then returning to damage the public's health.

Today, this concern has been exemplified numerous times over by persistent pollutants along with metals and other toxicants. These include the polychlorinated biphenyls (PCBs), polybrominated flame-retardants (PBDEs), lead, and various pesticides, including DDT. The chemically stable perfluorinated compounds (perfluorooctanoic acid; PFOA or C8) that we met in the introduction did not exist a century ago but are now found worldwide and in virtually all Americans.[40] Short-lived substances such as bisphenol A (BPA) and phthalates are ubiquitous (because of enormous production) and toxic. BPA hardens plastics for containers and cases for electronics, along with many other uses. Phthalates are ingredients in shampoos, food packaging, perfumes, hairsprays, and cosmetics, but also soften plastics for intravenous lines and baby pacifiers.

By 1970 the accumulation of publicly visible adverse events and known toxicants in the environment, highlighted by *Silent Spring*, led to the first Earth Day. Millions supported protecting the Earth and its human, animal, and plant residents at this largest organized celebration up to that time. Following Earth Day, many major environmental and public health laws poured out of Congress. This was an extraordinarily productive legislative rate viewed from today's vantage of little federal legislation in the public interest. From 1970 to 1980 and a bit beyond, several Congresses passed dozens, possibly hundreds, of bills to clean up the environment and better protect the public from risks that could arise from chemical creations in consumer products, workplaces, food, and the environment, and from pollutants in the air, water, and soil.

President Richard M. Nixon, a conservative Republican, signed off on many of these laws passed by a Democratic Congress. Democratic senator Edmund Muskie, running for president and advocating protections for the environment and the public's health, likely assisted President Nixon's motivation.

As Congress enacted this legislation, it was aware of different models for how science and law could be utilized to protect the public. Legislators had choices about *when* in the life of a chemical creation that scientific studies should be used in environmental-health laws to protect the public. Congress was in effect choosing what kind of protection from chemical product to provide for the public. Unfortunately, for the vast majority of chemical creations in our midst, they passed numerous laws that create ignorance about our exposures (some of which are toxic), greatly delay improved health protections, and produce consequences that swamp discussions with a fog of science that likely confuses the public and sometimes administrators of the law.

ENVIRONMENTAL LAWS, 1970–1980

Federal laws are the main but not the only legislation providing environmental and environmental-health protections. Analogous legislation was enacted by various states, but I consider only major federal laws.

The Food and Drug Administration

Two laws of note under the administration of the Food and Drug Administration (FDA) were the Food, Drug, and Cosmetic Act (FDCA) (1906, amended in 1962) and the Federal Insecticide, Fungicide, and Rodenticide Act (FIFRA) (1948, amended in

1972). The 1962 FDCA amendments instituted premarket toxicity testing and approval for pharmaceuticals, while other amendments along with aspects of the FIFRA provided authority over pesticide residues on foods. Importantly, both laws require tests on the created drugs and pesticides before entering commerce, and in each case a panel of scientists must review the tests. I return to this class of legislation below.

The US Environmental Protection Agency

At the same time, Congress authorized the creation of the Environmental Protection Agency (EPA), created new laws to protect the environment, and brought a number of environmental offices and laws under its administration. These included the Clean Air Act (1970); the Clean Water Act (1972); the Marine Protection, Research, and Sanctuaries Act (1972); and the Safe Drinking Water Act (1976). A common theme was an effort to ensure that the air we breathe, the water we drink, and that the waters in rivers and off beaches are fishable and swimmable.

After passing this legislation, Congress realized the need for an inventory of hazardous substances, as well as procedures for tracking them from the cradle in which they were created to the grave in which they were safely disposed. It passed the Resource Conservation and Recovery Act in 1976.[41]

Although a number laws sought to clean up various media—air, water, and soil—and protect the public, Congress had not dealt with a long legacy of improperly disposed chemicals (as C8 was). Many of these had merely been dumped into the ground, rivers, or even the ocean, with the result that many migrated elsewhere into the environment and threatened the public's health or the larger environment. Perchlorate, a component of rocket fuel with a comparatively short safe life in rockets, was typically hosed into the ground, inter alia, when it became too unstable for fuel. It migrated into the groundwater and continues to contaminate drinking-water sources. Polychlorinated biphenyls, dumped into the Hudson River, pose problems even today. DDT was dumped into the ocean off the coast of Southern California and continues to leach from its grave. The realization of legacy toxic-waste dumps led to the law commonly known as "Superfund"—the Comprehensive Environmental Response, Compensation, and Liability Act (1981)—with later amendments in 1986.[42]

The Occupational Safety and Health Administration

Employees could be exposed to toxic substances in workplaces that create or use them in other products, but were even more poorly protected before 1970. For instance, DuPont employees were exposed to C8 beginning in the 1950s, with the toxicity of C8 identified as early as 1961 and evidence that it was accumulating in employees' bodies by 1978. One of the first laws passed in 1970 was the Occupational Safety and Health Act, motivated in large measure by concerns about workers exposed to the deadly substance asbestos.[43] Even today, workers continue to die from asbestos-caused diseases, but the apex of annual deaths has not yet been reached because of the latency period of this disease.[44] At the same time, Congress authorized the creation of the Occupational Safety and Health Administration (OSHA) to implement the law.

The Consumer Product Safety Commission

People could also be exposed via consumer products, paints, and various poisons. A new Consumer Product Safety Commission addressed these with authority to administer the Consumer Product

Safety Act (1972) and the Lead-Based Paint Poison Prevention Act (1973), to go with the earlier Federal Hazardous Substances Act (1960). During this burst of legislation, Congress passed other laws, but those mentioned above include the more important ones.

The need for more-comprehensive protections

In the early to mid-1970s, Congress realized that there was a need for a more comprehensive law governing the creation and safety of all chemical substances that were being produced. This was the Toxic Substances Control Act (TSCA). Because this law is central to understanding the regulatory protections for human health, I return to it below.

Legislation seeking to protect the public from toxic chemical creations (or pollutants) falls into two generic categories: premarket laws and postmarket laws. *Premarket* testing and scientific review laws seek to identify risks from products *before* they enter commerce and people are exposed.[45] Such laws notably govern pharmaceuticals and pesticides. Chemical creations must be routinely subjected to a specified battery of tests (different for each class of substances) and undergo independent scientific review at the appropriate administrative health agency—the FDA for pharmaceuticals or the EPA for pesticides—before they may be sold in the market. They then typically remain in the market until the agency bears a legal and scientific burden of proof sufficient to change their legal status to reduce or eliminate risks.

The 1976 TSCA, which has governed all the general chemicals currently in commerce, has a partial, but poor, premarket feature—a "notification" provision. Unlike pharmaceutical and pesticide laws, it does not *routinely require toxicity data about products before they enter commerce*. Rather, a company proposing to manufacture a chemical creation need only notify the EPA that it seeks to manufacture a product by submitting certain data about it. Given its import and provisions for environmental health protection, I develop its provisions more fully below.

Postmarket health laws do not legally require manufacturers of chemical products, or those who might have them in waste streams or who might use them or who might incorporate them into their products, to routinely test for and identify risks before they enter the environment and people are exposed. (Despite TSCA's premarket notification provision, I regard it as a postmarket law because no routine toxicity tests have been required of products before entering the market.) Once products are in commerce, they remain there until the EPA or other health agency has data showing they are toxic. Then it has a legal and scientific burden of proof that must be supported by sufficient data, resources, and political will in order to change the legal status quo to protect the public's health.

Postmarket laws seek to prevent health harms from occurring by identifying risks *after* products are in commerce and exposures have occurred or are likely to exist, but before risks materialize into harm or before too much harm is done. These laws govern environmental hazards from general chemical releases as well as pollutants and chemical creations in air, water, drinking water, waste sites, occupational settings, and consumer products.

Figure 1 provides a generic depiction of those laws.

THE INFLUENCE OF NUISANCE LAWS
ON ENVIRONMENTAL LAWS

"To a surprising degree, the legal history of environmental law has been written by nuisance law," according to William Rodgers, a

Generic Legal Strategies to Protect the Public Health

Postmarket laws	Premarket laws
Substances enter commerce/environment with *no legally* required routine toxicity testing or approval (~90–80% of all chemical creations)	Premarket toxicity testing and approval laws *legally require routine toxicity testing & agency approval* before products can enter commerce. These *mainly* govern pharmaceuticals and pesticides (~10–20% of all chemical creations).
	Pre-market *notification laws*—one aspect of the 1976 Toxic Substances Control Act. *No* required toxicity testing; only submission of what is known about a creation.

Figure 1 Generic legal strategies to protect the public health.

leading environmental law scholar.[46] Congress based many of the environmental and public health laws on what we might call postexposure, postviolation nuisance laws. Nuisance laws historically were part of the tort or personal-injury law.

What are nuisances? These are activities or pollutants that could interfere "with the use or enjoyment of land, and . . . [were] the parent of the law of private nuisance as it stands today," but these also include public nuisances.[47] They include smoke, dust, unpleasant odors, excessive light from nearby structures, loud noises, or repeated and annoying phone calls, all of which might disturb a person's comfort or convenience.[48] A more public nuisance might be a "disagreeable stench, recognizable by anyone with a functioning nose, [which would] justify resort to the best techniques available to sweeten the air."[49] Other nuisances might include vibration, blasting, destruction of crops, flooding, pollution of a stream, or fear of contagion from tuberculosis.[50]

If citizens find "substantial and unreasonable interferences" with land or the public that are "offensive or inconvenient to a normal person," they may bring a legal action (sue) in torts for compensation or to stop the nuisance with an injunction. To do so a person must make a *postexposure, postviolation* showing of substantial and unreasonable interferences with her land, as judged by a normal person in the area. She must file a case in the tort law after a nuisance occurs. She must also have evidence of the interference and harm, typically straightforward for the vast majority of quite detectable nuisances.[51]

Antipollution laws were at the head of the congressional queue in the 1970s because many environmental problems that led to the first Earth Day were visible pollutants, not unlike nuisances. Nuisance law was an especially apt and well-understood model for pollution laws such as the Clean Air Act (CAA) and the Clean Water Act (CWA) that aimed to cleanse burning rivers or clear polluted air. Before there were environmental health administrative agencies, alleging a nuisance was a legal route for addressing obvious pollutants and their consequences.

About the same time, Congress realized that existing legislation targeting different media—the air, soil, rivers, harbors, and drinking water—would fail to address myriad new and existing chemical substances and would be poorly governed by media based laws. They would likely have to be approached, not in a unified manner, but on a cumbersome media-by-media basis. And any harmful substances would likely be toxic in several different media. Thus, it sought a uniform law to govern all commercial chemicals at the time of creation.

While nuisance law provided one model for protecting people from chemical substances, the amended FDCA of 1962 provided a different model. These amendments resulted from the public health catastrophe caused by the poorly tested sedative Thalidomide.

This pharmaceutical was typically prescribed to assist sleep and to calm nerves. However, the American licensee, Richardson-Merrell Pharmaceutical, seeking to increase its sales, advertised it "to treat the nausea of early pregnancy."[52] The campaign worked; some pregnant women chose thalidomide to ameliorate morning sickness and other upsets during the first trimester of pregnancy. During this critical period, a developing child's organs, its limbs in particular, begin to emerge. Among women who took thalidomide 5000–7000 mothers gave birth to babies with shortened limbs. These newborns also exhibited a host of other adverse effects, including neurological problems, deformed spines, heart disease, sometimes missing ears or eyeballs, kidney abnormalities, and autism, to name just a few. In addition, another 7000–8000 babies aborted or were stillborn.[53] Importantly, because a skeptical young scientist at the FDA, Francis Oldham Kelsey, resisted the approval of thalidomide because of poor safety data, Americans were better protected, with about 40 thalidomide babies born in the United States.[54]

This worldwide disaster made clear to Congress that chemical substances could cause adverse effects in children in utero during their development. Consequently, the Democratic Senator Estes Kefauver working on other amendments to the FDCA included a provision to require premarket testing and scientific review of the tests *before* a pharmaceutical would be approved for sale. Despite initial and nearly unanimous opposition by Republicans led by Richard M. Nixon, the amendments unanimously passed both the Senate and the House of Representatives in 1962. What congressman wanted to be in favor of deformed babies?[55]

These amendments for pharmaceuticals represented an alternative model for addressing the toxicity of chemical creations at the point of manufacture. The President's Council on Environmental Quality (CEQ) in 1971 clearly understood this: toxic substances were entering the environment, they could have severe effects, and existing legal authorities were inadequate to address toxicity as these substances were being created. Consequently, it recommended that Congress write a law to address these issues. At the same time, experience with the persistent and quite toxic PCBs reminded decision makers that chemicals not used as pesticides "were not yet covered effectively by any existing law." PCBs caused hazards for ecosystems and communities around the world, including poisonings.[56]

This also helped motivate CEQ's concern to identify toxic substances before they entered the environment and before people were exposed.[57]

> We should no longer be limited to repairing the damage after it has been done [a reference to the tort law]; nor should we continue to allow the entire population or the entire environment to be used as a laboratory [as had occurred under some laws].[58]

It endorsed premarket testing of all chemicals entering commerce: "A new substance (excluding products covered by other regulatory authority) could be marketed only after it met [various test] standards."[59]

Thus, as Congress considered legislation for chemical creations at the point of manufacture to protect the public from potentially toxic substances, it had two models: postexposure, postviolation analogues to nuisance laws and the premarket toxicity testing and scientific review laws Congress had recently enacted for pharmaceuticals and then pesticides.

The CEQ, the Nixon administration, and the members of congress sponsoring of the law proposed a premarket-testing and scientific review law somewhat resembling premarket laws for pharmaceuticals and pesticides. However, as it went through the legislative process, environmentalists "only mildly supported" this proposal; they were more focused on "the clean air and water bills." Industry strongly opposed premarket-testing provisions.[60] In 1976, after a five-year effort, Congress passed the TSCA. Premarket toxicity testing lost.

With this choice, one might say that Congress put Jeromy Darling, Ken Wamsley, Carla Bartlett, and Sandy Guest at greater risk than they might have been under a premarket toxicity testing law. The life-threatening diseases that they contracted might have been prevented had the toxicity of C8 and formaldehyde been detected under a different federal law. We have seen how they were affected.

Were many in Congress so focused on laws to control largely *detectable environmental invaders,* typical of some obvious environmental problems, that they did not realize many issues that could arise from toxic substances? Were they unaware of how biologically active and toxic general chemicals could be (as researchers have now discovered)?[61] Did the chemical industry's intensive lobbying move Congress away from a premarket testing and scientific review law overwhelm all other efforts? Given competing models that could have influenced its legal structure, what are some of its main provisions?

THE RESULTING TOXIC SUBSTANCES CONTROL ACT

As already noted the Lautenberg Act just amended the 1976 TSCA. Some amendments correspond to recommendations that others and I have suggested over many years. Yet in this chapter I discuss the effects of the 1976 law because of its long-term influence.

All current general chemicals in commerce, considered "new" or "grandfathered" in the past, have been subject to this legislation and we should understand the problems this has created. Under the Lautenberg Act, even with some improvements, many challenges discussed in this chapter and chapter 4 will continue to hamper public health protections for years to come. In that chapter I discuss some strengths and continuing shortcomings of the Lautenberg Act.

First, the 1976 TSCA governed the overwhelming percentage of all existing and new chemical creations from 1976 to the present.[62] Second, for *existing* chemicals at the time, TSCA grandfathered as "safe" an inventory of about 62,000 "general" substances manufactured or imported into the United States (1979), excluding comparatively small numbers of prescription drugs, pesticides, tobacco products, nuclear material, foods, new food additives, chemical mixtures, and cosmetic ingredients.[63] C8, formaldehyde, and the PBDE flame retardants were on this list. Third, any substances not on the initial inventory would be considered "new." These would be subject to a premanufacture notification (PMN) requirement. After the EPA has approved new chemicals to be manufactured under a PMN submitted by companies, these chemicals would be added to the inventory and could be manufactured.

Unlike the legal requirements for pharmaceuticals, new chemicals do not undergo legally required routine toxicity tests. The PMN provision for all new chemicals or for substantial new uses of existing substances is a small but inadequate gesture toward identifying the toxicity of chemicals before public exposures occur.

A PMN for submitted substances must be accompanied by "all available data on chemical identity, production volume, byproducts, use, environmental release, disposal practices, and human exposures."[64] This language requires no toxicity data for new products. If a company has conducted any toxicity tests, it is legally required to submit them, but if it has not, there is nothing to submit. The EPA "must take what it is given."[65] As a result roughly "33% of PMN submissions include some test data on the chemical properties, . . . [but only about] 15% of submissions include data on health effects." About 85% lack health data.[66]

At the time, many hoped (and the legislative history presumed) "that [voluntary] testing of new products would take place before they were widely used . . . [although] TSCA forbids promulgation of blanket testing requirements for all new chemicals . . ."[67] This voluntary option has not been taken, and in fact many companies ceased testing their creations at all. The Congressional Research Service finds that "most existing chemicals still lack toxicity data relevant to hazard assessment."[68] I return to this below.

Since 1980, about 22,000 substances have been added to the chemical inventory, out of about 44,000 PMNs submitted.[69] (Not all proposed substances are developed, and some are voluntarily withdrawn.) In 2009 the TSCA inventory was about 84,000 registered for commerce.[70]

Unfortunately, and quite importantly, the law requires *no* routine *toxicity* or *health effects data* before a product is commercialized. The EPA may require toxicity data about a proposed chemical product, but only if there is evidence that it poses "unreasonable risks" to public health or the environment. If the EPA has the pertinent evidence, it may "issue a regulatory rule" ordering the information.[71]

However, the agency must have data "to prove that it needs it, but it needs the information because it does not have it," a catch-22 situation.[72] Moreover, even if it has enough minimal information legally to compel further studies by the company, it must issue a legal order for the tests, which requires substantial time, resources, and personnel to carry out. Eventually, because of the difficulties and burdens of requiring further testing, the EPA developed a program of voluntary compliance that has led to somewhat more testing.[73]

Despite the PMN provision for new products, the 1976 TSCA largely functions like a postmarket law. There are no necessary assurances of safety for new products (with little or no toxicity testing) or products grandfathered as safe; thus, little is typically known about them. And there is no mandatory review of existing chemicals in commerce.[74] This is similar to nuisances before they become noticed. Once chemical creations are in commerce, if scientists find that they pose risks, they are treated as a postmarket, postexposure, postviolation enforcement issue.

Yet, nuisances suffer deep dissimilarities with toxic molecules. Laws that can reasonably govern nuisances are greatly flawed for addressing tiny, undetectable substances whose toxic effects are often delayed. Nuisances typically signal clear evidence of their presence and interference with others' interests, in contrast to toxic molecules such as benzene, lead, PCBs, or PBDEs. Have you ever "seen" or detected any of these molecular substances? However, you likely have been aware of or have experienced some typical nuisances. How scientists could identify and discover adverse health or environmental effects from molecular invaders poses much more substantial barriers than nuisances, since the causal effects of molecules are critically more difficult to discern.[75]

Congress may have failed to understand the difficulties of identifying toxic molecules and their causal effects (compared with nuisances) in order to protect the public. Because nuisances are readily apparent through our sight, hearing, smell, taste, touch, or ability to detect vibrations, typically we need not rely on scientific studies to determine that nuisances are present or perhaps even how serious they are.

In contrast, chemical creations can sneak up on someone, entering his or her body via drinking water, the air, or food and initiating biological processes that cause harm, but the person is none the wiser. Carla Bartlett was unaware her drinking water would lead to kidney cancer. Sandy Guest surely did not know that Brazilian Blowout contained formaldehyde or that it could cause leukemia and kill her. Our senses are largely useless for discovering them or their causal effects. Thus, for scientists to determine whether nonpharmaceutical, nonpesticidal chemical creations are invading and have the potential to cause harm, they need subtler and more technical tools than ordinary senses.

SHORTCOMINGS OF TSCA AND OTHER POSTMARKET LAWS

The postmarket legal regime for protecting the public from potential toxicants, with a most important role by the 1976 TSCA, generates numerous problems. The law itself has created considerable ignorance about existing and new chemicals. It also encouraged willful obliviousness about chemical products, permitted risks and potential harms, and created barriers to better health protections. Even wise, conscientious, and well-motivated scientists committed to protecting the public's health must start from near total knowledge gaps about a substance's toxicity in order to generate data aimed at reducing risks or removing the substance from commerce. It consequently makes haphazard guinea pigs of adults and children alike (chapter 2). Finally, because it is a postmarket enforcement law, companies have strong incentives to resist losing profit-generating products and are tempted to use all available means, honorable and less honorable, to serve these ends. Consider each issue in turn.

POSTMARKET LAWS CREATE AND INVITE WILLFUL IGNORANCE ABOUT CHEMICAL PRODUCTS

Legally created ignorance

TSCA codified considerable ignorance about the toxicity of products. Importantly, 75% of the current existing chemical creations were grandfathered as "safe." Why? Testing so many substances would have been quite burdensome and taken decades. Perhaps there was little overt evidence of toxicity among these substances. Maybe, at the time, general chemicals were not considered to be as biologically active in human bodies as pharmaceuticals were designed to be, and as pesticides were created to be in insects, weeds, and rodents. (Of course, this would have been contrary to the experience of PCB poisonings that occurred and contributed to the need for TSCA.) The 1979 presumption of the "safety" of general chemicals still holds and can be overcome only by showing that substances pose "unreasonable risks" to human health or the environment.

TSCA also made it difficult to reveal the toxicity of *new* chemicals that have little or no toxicity data. Companies may voluntarily choose to test (or not to test) any new substances and be in full compliance with the PMN requirement, but how well has this worked to protect the public? Not well, as I will argue.

Tempting willful ignorance

TSCA's 1976 new chemicals policy, by providing companies a choice to ascertain any adverse effects, gave them permission not to know of their products' toxicity. This in turn created avoidance and competitive incentives to be willfully ignorant of their new products.

If Company A tests a product but finds no toxic effects, it is presumptively free from legal requirements. However, if its tests show the substance is toxic, the company is required to report that result to the EPA. (It is clear that companies do not necessarily comply with the law.[76]) The agency in turn would then have some scientific data suggesting that the product "may pose an unreasonable risk to health or the environment," potentially triggering an EPA order for more test data. Such data would also be subject to discovery in the tort law. The company would have helped create additional testing and costs for itself or invited tort law suits, and perhaps more trouble! Consequently, before a company knew anything at all about its substance, from a self-interested and cost minimization point of view, should it conduct tests? Given these potential outcomes, why test? DuPont remained silent for years about toxic effects it found from C8.[77]

A company might engage in "innocent" or less innocent willful ignorance of risks from its products. Without any knowledge or clues about a product's toxicity, to which others would be exposed, putting its testing head in the sand like an ostrich would contravene important social responsibilities. Perhaps this might not rise to serious wrongdoing. However, the legal incentive is more pernicious if a company suspects a product may have toxic effects, but fails to test it. Not making "a reasonable inquiry" about the toxicity of a product would constitute "Deliberate avoidance . . . of [making] a reasonable inquiry about [toxicity]. . . ."[78] DuPont knew decades earlier that C8 was toxic to rats, dogs, and rabbits, killing some of them, with strong hints that it adversely affected their employees, but the company only quite belatedly reported this to the EPA.[79] Jeromy Darling's, Ken Wamsley's, Carla Barnett's, and Wilbur Tennant's cows' diseases were among the failures of these choices.

Competitive incentives also undermine voluntary testing. If Company A tests its products but Company B doesn't test its products, then Company A's cost structure is higher than Company B's. Consequently, both companies have competitive incentives not to test their products.

Unfortunately, this incentive structure likely motivated major chemical companies to eliminate their often quite good toxicology departments.[80] They intentionally chose to eliminate the means to determine the toxicity of their products and to remain ignorant about future product lines.

Resulting chemical ignorance

Quite substantial ignorance about the chemical universe resulted. In 1984 the National Research Council found

- 12,860 substances produced in excess of one million pounds/year (78% had no toxicity data) [postmarket].
- 13,911 chemicals of less than one million pounds/year (76% had no toxicity data) [postmarket].
- 8627 food additives (46% had no toxicity data) [partly postmarket].
- 1815 drugs (25% had no toxicity data) [premarket].
- 3410 cosmetics (56% no toxicity data) [postmarket].
- 3350 pesticides (36% no toxicity data) [premarket].
- 21,752 chemicals with production unknown or inaccessible (82% had no toxicity data) [likely postmarket].[81]

Postmarket laws governed the vast majority of the chemical creations shown above that lack toxicity data. This is what one would expect from TSCA's provisions and earlier laws requiring no testing.

Notably, two laws that by the early 1970s had premarket-testing provisions—pesticides and pharmaceuticals—had more products with better toxicity data than the general universe of substances. However, it is hardly impressive that 25% of pharmaceuticals and 36% of pesticides lacked toxicity data. Some of this is likely explicable by earlier "legacy" substances, that had not been tested for toxicity before premarket testing was required under each law.

In 1990 the National Research Council again consulted with members of the initial committee, seeking to update the 1984 report. But there was no new information with which to update the earlier study.[82] In 1997 the Environmental Defense Fund conducted a similar survey and found that about 70% of the substances still lacked toxicity data, not a major improvement from 1984.

In 1998 the US EPA, with urging from environmental organizations, created the High Production Volume (HPV) Challenge Program "to make health and environmental effects data publicly available on chemicals produced or imported in the United States in the greatest quantities." Initially, companies sponsored somewhat more than 2200 HPV chemicals.[83]

The HPV program has been the only systematic effort by the EPA to develop and foster "public access to basic hazard data on a relatively large number of chemicals in commerce." Despite its potential, it fell short. Companies sponsored only 1900 substances. One-third of those lacked final data sets, and 20% lacked even initial submissions of test results. Most of the chemicals were not directly tested for toxicity but instead used surrogates such as toxic estimations or structural similarities.[84]

Since 1980 the EPA itself has required testing of about 200 substances out of the 62,000 in commerce in 1979 (0.3 of 1%). Were the 61,800 remaining substances really "safe"? The General Accounting Office found that the EPA has "reviewed" only 2% of the 62,000 grandfathered substances, or a total of 1200.[85] Were the other 60,800 free from toxicity? Finally, the Congressional Research Service reports that the EPA has "rarely" imposed involuntary testing requirements on new substances; it is simply too burdensome.[86]

Companies could also shield their creations from public scrutiny by classifying them as "confidential business information (CBI)," a legal category permitted under TSCA to protect the value of products. About 90% of new chemicals were so classified.[87] Consequently, citizens had and continue to have even greater ignorance about the chemical universe and their exposures than public health agencies. (The CBI provision has been somewhat modified in 2016.)

Flame retardants: From grandfathered "safety" to ubiquitous invasions and diseases

One class of substances illustrates some of the problems: brominated flame retardants were grandfathered as safe in 1979. Created to retard flames, and provide more time to extinguish them, flame-retardants have been used in furniture, electronic devices, mattresses, upholstery, carpet pads, and baby seats, inter alia. In the mid-1970s, US citizens had no PBDEs in their bodies. If a company sought to create flame retardants for its products, it could do so because of their presumed safety.

If the company planned to greatly ramp up production, it would have to notify the EPA under TSCA's PMN provisions.[88] If the EPA obtained information indicating that PBDEs were toxic, it could require further data by issuing a rule or, perhaps, seek to have the company voluntarily provide needed data.

If the EPA took no action as production increased, a company could market the PBDEs in greater volume. If the company at some point became aware of toxic properties, it was legally obligated to report them. The public likely continued in ignorance about the toxicity of PBDEs.

Eventually, if scientists became concerned about the toxicity of PBDEs, they could seek funding to search for toxic properties. Efforts from individual researchers might not be coordinated, but each would aim to understand toxicity from her disciplinary perspective. If enough independently generated data alerted the EPA to the PBDEs' toxicity, the agency would have to determine whether they pose an "unreasonable risk" to human health or the environment.[89]

In 2017, US citizens now have the highest concentrations in the world of PBDEs in their bodies. While researchers understand some of their adverse effects from animal data, they are just beginning to identify toxic effects in people.[90] The PBDE flame retardants are endocrine disruptors, mimicking and displacing natural hormones. They are reproductive toxicants, delaying pregnancies in women with higher levels of PBDEs in their bodies. They are neurotoxic: children with higher PBDE exposures have impaired attention, lesser verbal and full-scale IQ, and deficiencies of fine motor coordination.[91] As children with substantial PBDE exposures develop, they may manifest other diseases or dysfunctions that have been presaged by animal studies. There are several major variants of PBDEs, but as yet there is no national ban on any of them; a few states have banned one variant and some have been phased out.[92]

Ignorance in the market

Ignorance about toxicants can cause health problems or prevent a market in less toxic products. Because so little is known about the universe of substances, ordinary citizens or companies may not know about the toxicity of a product to which they are exposed. If they seek to use less toxic products, they have little knowledge and fewer choices with different levels of toxicity. Consider three examples.

MCHM: Hundreds of thousands of West Virginians had their lives disrupted by the spilling of 4-methylcyclohexane methanol, or MCHM, into the Elk River source of their drinking water. Because of confidential business information, the amount produced in the United States is unknown. MCHM was grandfathered in 1979. There is utterly no authoritative hazard data available from governmental databases, including OSHA, the EPA, the National Institute of Occupational Safety and Health (NIOSH), or even the European Union.[93] Were West Virginians at risk of contracting life-threatening or non-life-threatening diseases? No one knows, and at present no one can know. Unless it is a quick-acting poison, which it is not, too little time has elapsed for many adverse effects to appear other than palpable minor irritations. However, some preliminary studies are beginning to show that MCHM is moderately toxic, and several of its metabolites are "related to genotoxicity due to its DNA damage effect on human cells and therefore warrants further chronic carcinogenesis evaluation."[94] Thus, the public cannot know about the potential toxicity of this product.

Oil dispersants: Similar toxic ignorance problems plagued oil dispersants used after British Petroleum's Deepwater Horizon explosion and oil spill in the Gulf of Mexico in 2010. The traditional oil dispersant that breaks large oil slicks into droplets was known to be toxic, at least for ecosystems. Immediately following the blowout, top EPA administrators asked their toxicologists about substitutes. There were some, but the agency could not choose between more toxic and less toxic dispersants.[95] The reason? Little or nothing is known about alternatives because of TSCA—they had either been grandfathered as safe or entered commerce with little or no toxicity testing. Early research is showing that the traditional dispersant causes damage to human lung cells and to the gills of fish and crabs. How serious is this? No one knows; only time will provide answers after appropriate scientific studies are reported.[96] In the meantime, fish, crabs, and humans are subject to a random experiment.

Bisphenol A: In recent years, BPA has been in the news for various possible and some actual harm it could cause. This endocrine-disrupting substance mimics the female hormone estrogen. BPA causes obesity in mice,[97] and it damages sperm production and causes breast cancer in rats, indicating it could cause similar effects in humans.[98] It may cause asthma in people[99] and possibly reduce control of impulsive behavior.[100] Other human studies suggest that "BPA is associated with increased risk for cardiovascular disease, miscarriages, decreased birth weight at term, breast and prostate cancer, reproductive and sexual dysfunctions, altered immune system activity, metabolic problems and diabetes in adults, and cognitive and behavioral development in young children."[101]

Because companies have been under considerable pressure to remove BPA from their products, some companies have replaced BPA with bisphenol S (BPS) or other substitutes. Unfortunately, academic researchers are now finding that BPS is more estrogenic than BPA.[102] So little is known about substitutes for BPA that an obvious alternative may be equally or more toxic. TSCA perpetuates this failure.

Back to C8: In 2009, DuPont replaced C8 with shorter-length molecules, presumably because they are safer. However, those substances are causing the same diseases in animal experiments that C8 did much earlier: "It's the same constellation of effects you see with PFOA," said Deborah Rice, a retired toxicologist who served as a senior risk assessor in the National Center for Environmental Assessment at the EPA. "There's no way you can call this a safe substitute."[103]

Because TSCA has led to considerable ignorance about substances, people who want choices between less toxic and more toxic products cannot have them because they do not have appropriate information.

BARRIERS TO BETTER HEALTH PROTECTIONS

Postmarket laws erect additional barriers to reducing risks and providing protections to the public. Because minimal or no scientific data are typically produced contemporaneously with commercialization of a product, research likely starts from scratch to determine any toxicity. This would have to be produced well after the creation entered the market and people have been exposed. Needed data would have to be accumulated from a minimal or no-data starting point.

Revealing any toxic effects can take considerable time because scientific studies march to their own drummers. Even if wise, conscientious, well-motivated scientists committed to protecting the public's health begin research as soon as toxicity is suspected, having cumulative results to support improved health standards can take substantial time.

However, as I argue later in this chapter, even when impartially and conscientiously developed science has been produced to protect the public, agency efforts have been hampered by companies' intransigence and by scientists who specialize in casting doubt on existing data, clogging protective efforts, leading portions of scientific fields astray, and greatly slowing improved public health protections. Moreover, efforts to cause doubt and slow health protections can create a "fog of science" that complicates public (and tort law) deliberations. Affected companies try to thicken this fog as much as possible to slow regulation. (Reducing risks from pharmaceuticals and pesticides requires similar processes, but these efforts do not seem quite as onerous as those under postmarket laws because initial studies provide the contours of chemical properties and some of their risks. They can also leave early clues about toxic properties that researchers can later discover. In addition adverse-reactions reports are available at least for pharmaceuticals.) Consider each of the above points in turn.

The theory for protecting the public under postmarket laws

How do laws governing substances already in commerce *prevent harm* if commercial products in fact are toxic? The answer lies in "risk assessment."

A risk is simply the chance or likelihood of adverse effects. However, just because there is a risk, this does not necessarily imply that anyone yet has been harmed. The hope for prevention of harm in a postexposure, postmarket context would use test results from nonhuman surrogates to reveal *risks* on which health agencies could quickly act to prevent health harms (or at least most harms) to the public. Surrogates could include whole-animal experimental trials, human cellular test tube data, bacterial data, mechanistic data, DNA information, and other tests. Thus, when public health agencies have sufficient data from surrogates to identify risks to humans, they can quickly reduce the risks before people are harmed.

Consider common but slightly elaborate risk assessment procedures as illustrative. If the EPA sought to know whether ambient water exposures of PFOA or C8 pose health risks, it would typically follow four generic steps:[104] hazard assessment, dose-response assessment, exposure assessment, and, finally, an overall risk characterization.[105] (Of course, at this late date and because company documents have revealed many known toxic endpoints of C8, this would be an easier task.)

First, is it a hazard? Can the agent in question cause an increase in the incidence of some adverse health condition? The adverse outcome might be a cancer, a reproductive disease, a neurological disorder, a lung disease, and so on.

Second, how potent is the substance? What concentration of the product will contribute to an adverse effect? Is the amount that causes adverse effects in parts per thousand, parts per million, or parts per billion?

Third, to what concentrations would people likely be exposed? What exposures would likely cause adverse effects?

Finally, how many people might be affected by the exposures? Would they contract life-threatening diseases, adverse effects leading to premature death, or perhaps only low-level and not serious adverse effects, or would they be subject to some combination of life-threatening and non-life-threatening risks?[106] For instance, recall that formaldehyde can cause burning eyes and sore throats along with several cancers.

Risk assessments are data intensive, providing full employment for experts from numerous disciplines. Complex scientific questions provide many opportunities for affected parties to object to the science, and because companies intransigently defend profitable product lines, they do so as long as possible.

Slow risk assessments

In 1987, the US Congress's Office of Technology Assessment found that each federal executive branch and independent agency responsible for reducing risks from carcinogens had only addressed 50% or fewer of the known carcinogens within its jurisdiction.[107] This occurred even though each agency or sub-office (e.g., the Safe Drinking Water Office within EPA) was working with presumptive data that the substances in question were likely to cause cancer to citizens.[108]

However, since that report, it appears that public health protections have been even slower, and thus the public is likely less well protected. Agencies are subject to substantial pressure to show human harm from exposures and to substantiate claims with multiple sources of data and multiple studies of each kind. All these increase the data intensiveness, which in turn increases the time that it takes to implement them. Improved health protections "become glacially mired in obfuscation, procrastination, and endless disputes about the science," delaying risk data on which to base health protections.[109]

Another indicator of this is the difficulty that the EPA has establishing even partial *risk estimates* through its Integrated Risk Information System, or IRIS (this is well short of a full health regulation). This involves only the first two steps of a typical risk assessment (above) but still proceeds slothfully (my term), reports the Governmental Accountability Office (GAO). Without risk estimates, the EPA cannot begin to go through other regulatory steps to protect the public by reducing or removing adverse effects.

TCE, a widely used solvent and metal degreaser, is a common environmental contaminant in air, soil, surface water, and groundwater. "TCE has been linked to cancer, including childhood cancer, and other significant health hazards, such as birth defects."[110] It also causes Parkinson's disease.[111] This substance has been awaiting a risk number for more than 20 years.

Dioxin, a byproduct of numerous industrial processes or a contaminant in some products, is a bioaccumulating human carcinogen (causing lymphomas and leukemia). It is a transgenerational toxicant and an endocrine disruptor widely contaminating the public through food, air, soil, plants, and water. It has been in the risk queue for more than 17 years.[112]

Perchloroethylene, used in dry cleaning and metal degreasing and in making some consumer products, is a probable human carcinogen and a common groundwater contaminant. It has been under review for more than 13 years.[113]

Formaldehyde, the human carcinogen we met in the introduction, which likely caused Sandy Guest's leukemia, also damages the respiratory system. One effort to provide a risk assessment had to be restarted because new data became available. A second effort to develop risk numbers for formaldehyde has been under review for 17 years and counting.[114]

Naphthalene, "used in jet fuel and in the production of widely used commercial products such as moth balls, dyes, insecticides, and plasticizers," is a probable human carcinogen that has been considered for more than nine years.[115]

The "quick risk assessment" theory has crumbled—likely based on a naive hope, founded on a flawed postmarket legal structure that incentivizes delays, and further eroded by the actions of lobbyists, corporations, and elected officials. Companies "game" the system, causing long delays.

FAILURES TO PROTECT THE PUBLIC

In addition to the above issues, since 1979 under TSCA the EPA has issued improved health protections for only five toxicants grandfathered as safe in 1979. Even to require testing of existing substances takes more than five years per compound to issue a regulation and longer yet to obtain test data.[116]

One major EPA attempt to eliminate all uses of asbestos under TSCA, with 45,000 pages of scientific and legal support, was vacated by the Fifth Circuit Court of Appeals. This extremely toxic substance could not be legally removed from the US market. What was the shortcoming? The "least intrusive" burden for asbestos brake linings was not considered, a requirement under the law.[117] The EPA has not used that TSCA provision again. If the agency cannot remove one of the most toxic substances from commerce under provisions from TSCA, what hope is there for protections from others?[118] In the 1970s some asbestos products were banned, but it can still be used in cement, clothing, roofing felt, vinyl floor tile, friction materials, disk brake pads, and gaskets, inter alia.[119] There is some good news for public health—thousands of successful tort suits have probably made it unprofitable to sell some products containing asbestos. Unfavorable publicity has also probably led consumers to avoid products that might have asbestos in them. California's Proposition 65 has long required warnings on products containing asbestos, likely discouraging some uses.

Despite all that is known about C8, the Teflon compound, there are still no national drinking water standards under the Safe Drinking Water Act (SDWA), even though C8 is present in many watercourses and drinking-water systems.[120] Sometimes public and perhaps legal pressures move companies to voluntarily withdraw their products from commerce, as DuPont has done with C8.

However, persistent substances in the environment can remain there and continue to invade and threaten the public's health.

As this book goes to press, the EPA has now issued a "Health Advisory" for C8. This is merely advisory to help managers of drinking-water systems protect the public. While it is based on "peer-reviewed science," it is not a legally enforceable federal standard under SDWA, which water systems across the country must follow.[121]

In addition to possible protective actions under TSCA, public health agencies may reduce exposures to toxicants under other laws. However, to do this they still need evidence of toxicity, ordinarily an assessment of their risks, and an affirmative regulatory determination to protect the public. Typically, toxicity data for most chemicals would be provided under provisions of TSCA, but other laws provide some routes by which substances can be identified as toxic and listed for public health protection. In addition, although many laws issue health regulations from lists of toxicants, some of these have been updated while others have been frozen in time. Currently, individual states have been able to set public health standards for toxic substances, if federal health agencies have not acted. However, under the Lautenberg Act that has just been enacted, states' legal authority will be more limited (chapter 4).

Consider how three subsidiary federal laws aim to protect the public.

The Clean Water Act (CWA) aims to keep toxic discharges from the nation's waters, such as rivers. Under this law the EPA has had a list of 129 toxic substances (resulting from a consent decree in federal court in 1978) for which there are limits for discharging them into rivers.[122] From this list the EPA develops national discharge standards for how much of each substance may be released into the nation's waters (if any at all). As of 1993 this list had not been updated, and that appears to remain true.[123] Thus, for example C8 is not listed even though it is highly toxic and has polluted numerous waterways. There is no nationwide standard restricting the discharge of C8 into rivers.

It is possible that Carla Bartlett's kidney cancer resulted from surface water contamination with C8 that had been "pooped" into rivers, as a DuPont lawyer put it. The surface water might well have become her drinking water. Since C8 was not regarded as toxic until fairly recently, there would have been no discharge limits on how much could go into surface water.

The SDWA authorizes the EPA to set "national primary drinking water regulation (NPDWR)" standards for contaminants in public water systems. Currently there are health protections for 90 contaminants in drinking water, which includes both inorganic (e.g., lead, mercury, beryllium, chromium) and organic (e.g., benzene, dioxin, PCBs, TCE, and vinyl chloride) toxicants.[124] C8 is not among them. The recent "advisory" (above) is an early step toward legally mandated health protections.

However, the EPA cannot issue an enforceable standard for C8 because it still lacks the needed risk numbers (more on this follows below). Managers of water systems likely will follow EPA's advisory document in order to better protect the public's health, but they are not legally required to do so.

The EPA can add to the drinking-water standards by taking them from a longer Contaminant Candidate List (CCL) and making a "regulatory determination" that there should be enforceable drinking-water standards. These listed substances are in or are likely to be in public water systems but are not "currently subject to EPA drinking water regulations."[125] The EPA can create regulations for a candidate contaminant provided that there is sufficient evidence that (1) it has "an adverse effect on the health of persons,"

(2) it occurs or has a high likelihood of occurring in public water systems often enough and at levels "of public health concern," and (3) regulation of the contaminant will likely result in "health risk reductions for persons served by public water systems."[126] The EPA is required to consider toxicants when updating the list every five years.

The EPA's IRIS, introduced earlier, would typically be the office that should conduct risk assessments for drinking water. However, we saw how slothful it has been in issuing risk numbers for formaldehyde and other substances. It has similarly been backed up in providing risk assessments needed under the SDWA. For instance, perchlorate, the poorly disposed-of rocket fuel component mentioned above, contaminates the drinking water of about 20 million residents in western US states, but there is no *national* drinking-water standard.[127] Some water systems have perchlorate concentrations in tens of thousands parts per million (10,000+ ppm). Compare this with California's drinking-water standard of 0.006 ppm (the concentrations in these western states are roughly 1.6 million times greater than California's safety standard).[128]

Under the CAA the EPA is also legally required to protect the public from hazardous (toxic) air pollutants. In 1990 Congress amended this law to require better health protections for 188 hazardous air pollutants (HAPs). For the first step the EPA was to issue standards for emission of these substances from sources of pollutants on the basis of the "maximum achievable technology."[129] After technology has reduced toxic air pollutant discharges to the extent it can, the EPA must then determine whether or not "residual risks" to the public health exist. For this, it needs risk data from IRIS. As of 2009, 20 years after Congress authorized these health protections, 17% of the HAPs were "not listed in IRIS at all," and two-thirds

(126 of the 188 on the congressional list) lacked important risk numbers to lower residual inhalation risks.[130] The public remains at some risk from these known toxicants.

What is the upshot of this brief discussion of less visible EPA offices for protecting the public's health? First, they need data that a substance is toxic from which the public should be protected. However, if it has not been identified as toxic under TSCA's burdensome procedures, how is it identified? Other EPA offices could identify it, but they may not be nimbly able to do so. Even if they know a compound is toxic, before they can actually issue legally enforceable protections, they have to follow other procedures under their authorizing statutes, which can take considerable time. Issuing better protections can also involve other parts of the EPA, such as IRIS, which can be a substantial hurdle. In most cases they must have risk data at certain concentrations of the toxicant in order to issue legally binding protections.

If these different health agencies have not acted and exposures to the public are high enough in drinking water or in the air, some people will not only be at risk, but will also be harmed. Postmarket laws and the conduct they invite make the protective steps much slower and more difficult (more in this chapter below).

Why are there delays and failures to protect the public?

Legitimate (excusable) and less legitimate reasons account for too little protection of the public. First, public health agencies must have *data* that a substance is toxic. If it does not have such data, nothing will happen. This may have been the case with DuPont's C8, since it was developed before TSCA was passed and the company kept its toxicity secret for many years. (However, once TSCA was enacted it would seem that DuPont could no longer use this reason.) Thus, companies have powerful incentives not to test their products (and equally powerful incentives to keep them secret, contrary to their legal obligations under TSCA).

Second, public health agencies have the burden of proof to reduce or remove risks. They must have information to assess the hazards, exposures, and ultimately the risks posed by products. Providing the requisite data takes considerable scientific investigation involving experts from many fields, as already noted.

Third, several different kinds of studies must be conducted and funded. Importantly, the studies have their own pace; they cannot be rushed. Human (epidemiological) studies must be of sufficient duration to reveal risks. There must be time for diseases to appear after exposures occur so that the diseases can be detected. (The fewer data that are initially available, the longer it takes.) Cancers can have latency periods from a few months up to 40 years. Parkinson's disease triggered early in life can remain hidden for several decades because a person's brain compensates for initial harm to the pertinent cells.

Without such data, there will likely be insufficient understanding of hazards and risks. Also, basing health protections on human studies requires that people have already contracted diseases for research to reveal. In order to protect other people, some must already have been ill! In the alternative, studies could be conducted on animals in order to estimate risks to people, but these can take up to seven years.[131]

Fourth, postmarket legal structures contribute substantially to delays. Because there would typically be little interest in substances until they are in the market, studies investigating their risks would ordinarily begin only after commercialization, as scientists begin to suspect their toxicity. Researchers begin with considerable ignorance.

Fifth, because public health agencies *have the burden of proof* to initiate action and to establish appropriate health standards to protect the public, those opposed need only resist, use blocking strategies, and play defense. The agencies have to make a sufficient scientific and legal case to reduce risks or remove the product from commerce. In contrast, affected companies have to argue only that the protective action has not been adequately established. Because products are in commerce generating income, companies have powerful incentives to oppose reduction of risks or removal of products. Often they urge that the very best or ideal science should support legal actions, and they portray themselves as scientific angels, which will help keep products in commerce longer (more on this in chapter 4).[132] They have also adopted less angelic strategies.

Creating scientific doubt with a fog of science

Affected companies and industry groups, protecting their products, have developed identifiable patterns using legal procedures under public health laws to slow improved postmarket health protections. They follow the lead of the tobacco industry: "Doubt is our product since it is the best means of competing with the 'body of fact' that exists in the minds of the general public. It is also the means of establishing a controversy."[133] Consistent with this, some companies claim to support the ideal of protecting the public, but they argue "at the moment" that the science is "too doubtful" (or perhaps not sufficiently "ideal" (chapter 4)) to support legal action. However, the moment just drags on and on and on. They generate a fog of (often misleading) scientific studies, trying to contradict or create doubt about impartially established findings, to reinforce uncertainty, to slow protections, and to keep their products in the market.

A typical pattern is that these companies attack early drafts of health assessments when public health agencies are required to post them. Then they force new reviews. Next, they hold workshops on the proposal populated with industry-funded panelists. Subsequently, they might introduce new industry-funded studies or industry-favorable interpretations of existing studies when public health protections are nearly final, which agencies must take into account.[134] After those are incorporated, an industry may try to force more reviews, all to slow the process. Before the process is over, they may enlist key politicians with political leverage. For instance, Senator David Vitter delayed the formaldehyde assessment for at least two years by holding President Obama's administrative appointments hostage in the US Senate until the he agreed to have its formaldehyde regulation reviewed by the National Academy of Sciences (NAS). This was in the interests of the best science, of course. (The NAS reported that the EPA correctly found that formaldehyde causes three different cancers in people, the main point of contention.[135]) Once that was completed the EPA might have to update or modify its assessment. When the EPA prepares to issue a final assessment, the affected industry might well start the process anew.[136]

The Center for Public Integrity reports that "Activity at the Environmental Protection Agency office that issues scientific reports on the toxicity of chemicals has nearly ground to a halt in recent years. . . . The agency faces intense pressure from Congress and industry whenever it determines that a chemical poses a greater risk to public health than previously thought. Industry hires scientists who argue that known carcinogens such as arsenic, formaldehyde, and hexavalent chromium are generally safe at currently allowable levels. The scrutiny has made it difficult for the EPA to update chemical regulations."[137]

We should note that legally mandated administrative procedures, created by Congress, are not innocent in delaying health protections. Agencies must follow the required law or face legal action for not doing so. Often, such procedures require them to use the best available evidence, and if quite recent tests are presented for consideration just as health protections are about to be issued, they must take them into account.[138]

There are no national public health standards for formaldehyde because of such strategies. People are still exposed. Some have become sick and others may have died, as Sandy Guest did. We may never know the full consequences of such delays because there is likely little motivation to generate the difficult but needed science to document the consequences. As a result, great delays can cause more harm, but no responsible party may be identified.

Less honorable tactics

Much-worse approaches were developed using the tobacco industry's strategies to frustrate health protections.

Many studies have found that who pays for studies can affect what they show. Sheldon Krimsky, an expert on research ethics, reports, "[T]here is sufficient evidence in drug efficacy and safety studies to conclude that the funding effect is real. Industry-sponsored trials are more likely than trials sponsored by nonprofit organizations, including government agencies, to yield results that are consistent with the sponsor's commercial interests." Over a wider range of studies, "bias [in studies supported by companies or industries] may exist." For direct tobacco smoke and secondhand tobacco smoke, industry "research shows a clear demarcation between studies funded by the cigarette industry and studies funded by nonprofit and governmental organizations.... [T]obacco industry ... scientists [played] a similar role as their contracted lawyers, namely, to develop a brief, in this case a scientific argument, that provides the best case for their interest."[139]

Recent investigative reporting suggests the spread of such strategies. Asbestos, used in brake linings, has been identified by numerous independent scientific organizations as causing mesothelioma (and other diseases) in mechanics and "backyard repairmen" who work on them.[140] After losing some tort law suits, in 2001 Ford Motor Company funded studies to "reshape asbestos science." It hired a scientist, Dennis Paustenbach, who is well known for finding industry-favorable scientific results.[141] The Center for Public Integrity reports that "Ford has spent nearly $40 million funding journal articles and expert testimony concluding there is no evidence brake mechanics are at increased risk of developing mesothelioma, ... an attempt at scientific misdirection aimed at extricating Ford from law suits, critics say."[142] They claimed that previous impartial science was mistaken. However, despite the effort to provide studies for favorable testimony in legal cases,

> "[T]hey've really produced no new science," said John Dement, a professor in Duke University's Division of Occupational and Environmental Medicine and an asbestos researcher for more than four decades. "Fifteen years ago, I thought the issue of asbestos risk assessment was pretty much defined. All they've accomplished is to try to generate doubt where, really, little doubt existed."[143]

The Ford effort seems particularly insidious and hypocritical because it chose to publish studies contradicting its own research. A 1986 memo reveals it knew of the risks of airborne asbestos fibers from brake linings. It knew that asbestos was in brake linings, that its fibers were "nearly indestructible, and [that] a potential health risk arises whenever fibers are set free resulting in airborne asbestos dust . . . [that causes] lung cancer and mesothelioma of peritoneum and pleura (cancer of the membranous lining of abdominal and chest cavities) . . . associated with asbestos inhalation."[144] Yet, 15 years later, the company sought to contradict well-established findings—including its own research—about the dangers of asbestos for science, the public, and legal venues. It apparently had some success in reducing tort suits from brake-lining exposures.[145] Did wrongfully injured mechanics go uncompensated? Are backyard mechanics still at risk?

Companies have had some success because they can hire experts to mislead public health agencies and subfields of science by publishing biased studies. As this book goes to press, the Center for Public Integrity has identified a number of scientists, companies that they have created, and journals in which they publish to present scientific studies contrary to university, nonprofit, and consensus scientific conclusions. These "scientists for hire" are favorable to companies that pay for their expertise and fund their work.[146] A number of scientists have long been known for conducting biased science on the fringes of disciplines or even outside them, according to academic researchers.

Less honorable tactics can be even worse. Sometimes, scientists or their employers have modified studies showing adverse effects in order to show that there are no, fewer, or lower risks from their products. For instance, the chromium industry began an epidemiological study of four newer industrial plants in order to assess any risks to employees. After preliminary results came in, researchers, apparently not liking the outcome, divided the study into two smaller studies, reporting results for two plants in one study and for two plants in another. Statistically this ensured there would be greater difficulty in detecting risks that were present (more on this in chapter 4). They could now present evidence that employees were at lesser risks from lung cancers than the original study revealed.[147]

However, David Michaels, then the assistant secretary for Environment, Safety, and Health in the Department of Energy, obtained the original study before it had been "reanalyzed." It showed that employees with intermediate exposures had a lung cancer risk five times higher than those in the lowest exposure group. The most exposed group showed a 20 times higher lung disease rate. For comparison, smokers inhaling a pack of cigarettes per day have a lung cancer rate about 10 times higher than nonsmokers.[148] Thus, it seems twice as safe to smoke a pack of cigarettes per day for a lifetime compared with a lifetime of work in the highest-exposed areas of a chromium plant!

In the same spirit, Merck Pharmaceutical, manufacturer of the pain medication Vioxx, seeking to show its benefits compared with a competitor, naproxen (Aleve), and to keep in the market, had study results showing that "Participants who took their drug for an average of nine months had *four times* the risk of heart attack as those taking Aleve [emphasis in original]."[149] Turning the results on its head, Merck argued that Aleve *lowered* the rate of heart attacks, an implausible result given earlier studies. Concerned about the outcome of the study, general suspicions by independent scientists, and skepticism at the FDA, Merck carried out a four-year rear-guard action. It sought to mislead physicians about the risks of Vioxx, attacked detractors, and "threatened the careers of academic physicians who questioned Merck's position on the safety of its drug."[150] It requested of Harvard researchers, who found that Vioxx increased the chances "of heart attacks compared with Celebrex or no related painkiller at all," to modify their conclusions. They refused.[151] Documents from litigation "show that its [Merck's] top scientists were worried about heart risks from Vioxx, and considered and rejected conducting specific studies to examine those risks."[152] In sum, "It is now clear that the correct interpretation of the Vioxx clinical trial was that the drug is a powerful cause of heart attacks. . . ."[153] Tens of thousands of preventable heart attacks occurred while Vioxx was in the market and during its delay from being withdrawn.[154]

While the Vioxx example shows that less honorable tactics are not restricted to products governed by postmarket laws, under premarket testing laws public health agencies and independent researchers begin their inquiries with more and better data. In addition, the pharmaceutical laws require companies and physicians to submit adverse-event reports, producing early warnings of potential adverse effects. Should researchers become concerned about toxic effects, they can return to existing premarket data and to adverse event reports, often finding clues to toxic effects that might have been missed earlier.

There are other examples, but I only reference them. (1) For perhaps 25 years, DuPont did not report known adverse effects from C8 identified in animal studies or adverse effects appearing in their employees.[155] (2) A surgeon, who specialized in treating burn victims, especially children, misled or even outright lied to legislators concerning the benefits of PBDE flame retardants.[156] (3) The American Petroleum Institute (API) funded studies of benzene in China that were marketed to find preordained results for its company supporters. Those seeking funding reassured potential funders that study results would require no changes in occupational exposures and that they would ease defending benzene in tort litigation.[157] They seemed to know the results of studies before they were ever conducted. (4) Lawyers have sometimes "ghostwritten" drafts of "scientific" articles needed for legal purposes and then solicited scientists to sign on to the paper.[158]

(5) A clearly furious state appellate judge reviewed an egregious example from the Bendectin litigation:

Studies for publication in peer review journals were tailored to the needs of litigation, and paid for out of defense funds. Most significantly, for the integrity of a judicial system, "scientific" articles for publication in "peer review" journals were edited before publication by lawyers litigating the issues presented in the article. The testimony revealed that "follow-up" studies were solicited by the defendant through intermediaries, funded by the defendants: but the scientific methodology changed, to obscure positive findings.[159]

Because practices such as these posed such a threat to the integrity of scientific research, editors of many medical journals demanded "that journals impose tougher disclosure policies for academic authors" and that they more actively investigate "the provenance of manuscripts and punish authors who play down extensive contributions by ghostwriters."[160]

(6) After 50 years of evidence had been developed about the toxicity of tobacco smoke, federal Judge Gladys Kessler in a legal ruling summarized the government's assessment of the tobacco industry's colossal efforts to protect their products.

[The various companies] have falsely and fraudulently denied: (1) that smoking causes lung cancer and emphysema as well as many other types of cancer; (2) that environmental tobacco smoke causes lung cancer and endangers the respiratory and auditory systems of children; (3) that nicotine is a highly addictive drug which they manipulated in order to sustain addiction; (4) that they marketed and promoted low tar / light cigarettes as less harmful when in fact they were not; (5) that they intentionally marketed to young people under the age of twenty-one and denied doing so; and (6) that they concealed evidence, destroyed documents, and abused the attorney-client privilege to prevent the public from knowing about the dangers of smoking and to protect the industry from adverse litigation results."

Moreover, her "Findings of Fact demonstrate that there is overwhelming evidence to support most of the Government's allegations."[161]

There is a deep irony from the above efforts. Frequently, industry groups argue that health protections should be based on "good, objective science," the Holy Grail to guide public policy. This especially occurs when scientific findings threaten their products.

Yet, many of the same groups seem to have tried to lead some subfields astray, skew the science away from objectivity and toward their views, and corrupt science. They published highly misleading studies or science known to be mistaken simply to protect their commercial products. The "ethics" of commerce took precedence over the public, public health agencies, judges, and other scientists. The chromium industry sought to show airborne chromium was safer than in fact it is. Asbestos companies hid the lethal effects of asbestos for decades while reaping commercial benefits.[162]

CONCLUSION

The CEQ, supporting toxicity testing at the point of manufacture, urged, "We should no longer be limited to repairing the damage after it has been done; nor should we continue to allow the entire population or the entire environment to be used as a laboratory."[163] Unfortunately, this is precisely where we are 45 years later and after the spate of 1970s environmental health laws. Postmarket laws have contributed to some progress—cleaning up rivers, harbors, the air, and drinking water—but much more remains to be done, as frequent news reports remind us. Some toxicants in commerce have been reduced or removed.

However, the language, structure, and incentives of the 1976 TSCA and other postmarket laws created substantial barriers to protecting the public's health. General ignorance about the toxicity of chemical creations, the slow pace of impartial science to identify toxicants, and companies' protection of commercial products by resisting public health protections and distorting the scientific literature leave the public at risk. It is likely that Jeromy Darling, Ken Wamsley, and Sandy Guest suffered serious diseases (or death in Guest's case) as a result of the ineffectiveness of these laws.

Providing sufficient data to reduce risks is delayed because even wise, conscientious, and well-motivated scientists committed to protecting the public's health start from scratch with minimal or no data. They must await the outcome of studies that proceed at their own pace.

Once studies reveal toxic risks sufficient to trigger improved health protections, companies fight to keep profitable products in the market. Honorably and less honorably they resist public health protections. The public bears the costs of ignorance and becomes involuntary, random guinea pigs for risky substances. When health harms occur, this is tragic.

When companies conduct or pay for misleading research that frustrates better health protections and continues health harms, tragedies for those harmed are enhanced because they need not have occurred. Yet, such misfortunes were knowingly instigated in order to frustrate, slow, or bar altogether legal actions seeking to protect citizens.

When decision makers knowingly mislead scientific fields and frustrate improved health protections, what might their reactions be? I do not know. However, since they often achieved their goals, this more than likely would be rewarding, not a matter of regret. Many who were hired to carry out such tasks also likely profited, often immensely (in millions of dollars), from their scientific roles.[164]

The harm occurring to citizens is not merely of historical or hypothetical concern. Increasingly research is finding that children during their development are much more susceptible to any toxic exposures than adults, and untold numbers of them have suffered harm as a result. This increases the urgency to reform postmarket laws and reduce toxicants in our midst.

Chapter 2

Cancers, Brain Disorders, and the Feminization of Boys

Can We Avoid Poisoning Our Children?

INTRODUCTION

Infectious diseases, caused by bacteria, viruses, fungi, or parasites,[165] are a leading cause of disability and death worldwide.[166] However, as they have declined dramatically in industrialized countries because of public health efforts, other diseases have risen in prominence. In developed countries, noninfectious diseases due to "environmental factors or gene-environment interactions"—cardiovascular disease, diabetes, obesity, respiratory ailments, and injuries—are on the rise and increasingly common.[167] Additional noninfectious diseases of concern include lead poisoning, childhood cancer, asthma, and brain disorders (e.g., attention-deficit hyperactivity disorder, dyslexia, autism, and other kinds of intellectual disability), along with immune system dysfunctions and reproductive disorders, such as the feminization of boys.[168] Recent research into the developmental origins of health and disease reveals numerous maladies and points to their sources.

This chapter adds substantial urgency to the concerns of chapter 1 by considering further consequences of laws that create and invite ignorance about chemical creations, some of which poison our children and the rest of us. Current postmarket laws cannot protect children as they develop from embryos to adults. The developmental period is one during which humans and other mammals are most susceptible to toxic exposures and other perturbations of their biology, although old age could be an important competitor.

Reducing exposures of children to toxicants has substantial importance because of their vulnerability and because they are exposed to a greater or lesser extent from conception onward. In addition, because young children have most of a full life ahead of them in which to be fully functioning, healthy people, on the one hand, or perhaps hampered by various diseases, disorders, and dysfunctions, on the other hand, this greatly adds to the concern. The following discussion reviews some of the biology of children during their development and considers some diseases that toxic substances can cause. It then argues that laws permitting such harms or threats of harm are unjust, and it sketches ways children can be better protected, which are developed further in chapter 4.

THE DEVELOPMENTAL ORIGINS OF DISEASE

What is the idea of the developmental origins of disease (or perhaps more accurately, the developmental origins of *health* and disease)? Generically, it is the theory that what happens to children during their development from embryonic and fetal life through infancy, early childhood, and the teenage years into adulthood can substantially influence their health and disease status, sometimes immediately but also even later in life. The full extent of these influences is currently not known because the science is in its infancy. However, research has demonstrated that both poor nutrition and exposure to toxic substances during this period of a human life can adversely affect a person's health.

Influences during the developmental period that perturb biological processes can result in numerous identified disorders that might appear at many periods of one's life. Disorders could include cardiovascular disease, obesity, type 2 diabetes and metabolic disturbances, immunological disorders, some forms of cancer and some neurological dysfunctions.[169] These effects can be subtle—they may or may not disrupt development or cause diseases themselves immediately—but may affect the rate at which disease develops in an individual.[170]

A canonic example showing how early-life influences can produce diseases much later in life resulted from a Nazi-imposed famine on the Dutch population in the winter of 1944–1945. During this "Dutch winter famine," adults received small food rations per day. For pregnant women this was inadequate to support the mother in good health, to say nothing of her developing child in utero. Consequently, undernourished pregnant women "deprived their developing children of adequate nutrition and calories in utero."[171] These children were often born with low birth weight. However, by then the Nazis had retreated, the famine had been lifted, and young children had more or less normal diets. Later, when a subset of these children reached the age of about 50 years, they showed "an increase in body weight, BMI [body mass index], and waist circumference. . . . Those low-birth-weight babies who were most vulnerable to developing obesity were men who had been light and thin at birth and had experienced a period of rapid childhood growth."[172] It was as if a biological message had been conveyed in utero that nutrition was scarce, so food resources should be utilized efficiently.

Indeed, famine-influenced newborns used food efficiently, typically showing "catch-up" weight gain. However, later in life they exhibited heart disease, diabetes, increased blood pressure, high blood sugar, abnormal cholesterol, and strokes, together called "the metabolic syndrome." This was programmed into them while they were developing in utero resulting in later-life diseases.[173]

This research has been replicated in different human populations and has been supported by experiments in sheep,[174] whose gestation period closely resembles humans', providing an excellent model to test the hypothesis.[175]

In addition, "*in utero* or neonatal exposures to environmental toxicants" can "alter susceptibility to disease later in life [by affecting] the programming of tissue function that occurs during development."[176] This in turn can "lead to altered [structural] and/or functional character of the tissues, organs and systems," potentially triggering diseases, dysfunctions, or premature death.[177]

The mechanisms by which such diseases and dysfunctions are caused are likely to be several and are not fully clear at this time. However, epigenetic phenomena provide one clear mechanistic explanation. This results in "altered gene expression or altered protein regulation [not a change in the genetic sequence producing] . . . altered cell production and cell differentiation . . ."[178] Epigenetic changes do not modify one's genetic sequence, but they alter when genes are turned on or off.

Such changes can affect not only first-generation offspring, but also in some instances second- and third-generation descendants as well. Moreover, it appears that numerous epigenetic changes can be permanent.[179] Surprisingly, some of these changes can become imprinted in the germ cells and affect later generations, even great-grandchildren and beyond (more below).

CITIZENS ARE EXPOSED TO AND INVADED BY TOXICANTS

That citizens are exposed to toxicants is not surprising, given the large number of untested new chemicals and the even larger number grandfathered as safe.

Because researchers and public health officials knew that drugs were designed to be biologically active in humans and would be put directly into their bodies by pill, injection, or intravenous line, since 1962 pharmaceuticals have been tested for their toxicity before entering commerce. Similarly, citizens have some degree of awareness that they are exposed to pesticides from numerous sources. Because these are designed to be biologically active and disrupt the functioning of insects, fungi, and rodents, inter alia, and we are aware that they can enter our bodies, Congress also chose to test them for toxicity before they entered the market.

When Congress amended the pesticide law with the Food Quality Protection Act (1996), it was known that pesticides could be inhaled, ingested, or absorbed through the skin. Legislators recognized that "*[E]xposures to pesticides do not occur as single, isolated events, but rather as a series of sequential or concurrent events that may overlap or be linked in time and space*" (emphasis in original).[180] Thus, the EPA must conduct "*aggregate assessment*" assessing how a single chemical might enter people's bodies by multiple pathways and routes. This approach makes the EPA's exposure and risk assessments closer to those "*actually encountered by individuals in the real world*" (emphasis in original).[181]

In contrast, general chemical creations (sometimes I dub them "industrial chemicals") are not typically designed to be biologically active in any species, but in fact many are. The public may not be aware that they are exposed to general industrial chemicals by multiple routes, yet they are. Chemical substances, including toxic molecules, can invade humans via ingestion, inhalation, and absorption through the skin, pathways identical to pesticides.

We might absorb toxicants from the food we eat, food containers, drinking water, or cooking utensils, as well as contaminants from external environments (such as air, river water, and the soil), or from internal environments in which we work and live. We might inhale air pollutants, dust, fugitive pesticides, toxicants in the workplace, dust from flame retardants in furniture, and even coal-tar-based fumes from the sealants on parking lots (and even track them into our homes).[182] Existing houses can have substantial toxic residues to which new residents can be exposed. Detectable amounts of more than 400 chemical creations, including many chlorinated pesticides, were measured in houses along the US-Mexico border.[183]

Although we may not think about it, we can also absorb chemical creations through the skin. A typical route might be from jewelry made of lead or cadmium. Cosmetics often contain a number of toxicants that are poorly controlled—phthalates, triclosan, etc. Some brands of lipstick contain lead, a notorious toxicant even at low concentrations.[184] An unusual chemical, methylphenyltetrahydropyridine (MPTP), was found to cause Parkinson's disease through ingestion and intravenously from illegal drugs. It also invaded a young chemist who worked with it in a laboratory through skin absorption and inhalation, causing Parkinson's-like symptoms.[185]

Citizens, including pregnant women, are contaminated by about 300 humanly created chemical substances that the Centers for Disease Control and Prevention (CDC) can reliably detect.

Some obvious contaminants include C8 in Teflon cookware, stain-resistant fabrics (including in sofas and carpets), food packaging, and Gore-Tex, now widespread in the environment; polybrominated flame retardants (PBDEs) in upholstery, plastic cases for electronic instruments, seat cushions, furniture, carpets, and draperies, as well as in the environment; polychlorinated biphenyls (PCBs) in foods, meats, the environment, air, and water; organochlorine pesticides; phthalates in cosmetics, linoleum flooring, and intravenous lines; polycyclic aromatic hydrocarbons (PAHs) from combustion; and perchlorate, a rocket fuel and fireworks component that is in groundwater, drinking water, and soil.

However, the above are probably just the tip of a contamination iceberg, especially since the vast majority of substances are untested for their toxicity. More commercial chemicals will be found in people's bodies because the CDC and some states, including California, are developing reliable protocols for identifying substances in blood and urine. Many are known or suspected toxic substances.[186]

Pregnant women are not immune to invasion, having up to 43 substances from 12 classes of compounds.[187] Some groups of compounds, including "polychlorinated biphenyls, organochlorine pesticides, PFCs, phenols, PBDEs, phthalates, polycyclic aromatic hydrocarbons, and perchlorate[have been] detected in 99–100% of pregnant women."[188]

This is especially worrisome because a pregnant woman's contamination is shared with developing children in utero.[189] There is "no placental barrier per se: the vast majority of chemicals given the pregnant animal (or woman) reach the fetus in significant concentrations soon after administration."[190] New technologies are joining the invasions: plastic nanoparticles can move from mom to baby through the placenta.[191]

Developing humans are at risk from toxicants from the moment of fertilization through embryonic and fetal life in utero. For instance, developing fetuses have near "universal exposure" to a substance such as bisphenol A (BPA), as do all adults, but fetuses have greater concentrations of free BPA (a more harmful variant) than are found in maternal blood or urine.[192] Umbilical cords of newborns, containing industrial chemicals, some toxic, reveal evidence of in utero exposures.[193]

After birth, children continue to be exposed to various chemical creations and pollutants (as all people are), but they are typically exposed at higher rates.[194] If we care about our children, as any parent, grandparent, relative, or ordinary citizen does, this greatly increases the urgency to protect them from toxic invasions.

DEVELOPING CHILDREN HAVE GREATER EXPOSURES THAN ADULTS

Developing children tend to be exposed to greater concentrations of chemical creations than the mother and adults more generally, whether in utero or after birth. In utero they tend to have larger doses of toxicants relative to their body weight than does the mother. For instance, mercury concentrations can be at least five times higher in the fetal brain than in the mother's blood.[195] Also, because children need calcium for their developing bones, a pregnant mother provides it via a "calcium stream" from her bones to theirs. If her bones contain lead, where it typically has a half-life of 25 years, it is mobilized and transferred to the developing child.[196]

Nursing newborns can also receive greater concentrations of toxicants. Lipophilic substances (fat loving), such as PCBs, are present in breast milk at much-higher concentrations than in the mother's blood serum. Some phthalates are concentrated five times greater in children than in adults, but, surprisingly, perfluorinated compounds (C8) are much lower in breast milk than in blood serum.[197] Scientists note that breast milk contamination is not a reason to refrain from breastfeeding, because on balance it is desirable, but newborns' contamination is worrisome.

DEVELOPING CHILDREN ARE MORE SUSCEPTIBLE TO DISEASES

Humans are quite vulnerable to toxic chemicals during early developmental stages. As the First International Conference on the Developmental Origins of Disease noted, "The periods of embryonic, fetal and infant development are remarkably susceptible to environmental hazards. Toxic exposures to chemical pollutants during these windows of increased susceptibility can cause disease and disability in infants, children and across the entire span of human life."[198] Developing children also "tend to be more sensitive to adverse environmental influences . . . [with] tissues undergoing rapid cell division."[199]

DEVELOPING CHILDREN HAVE LESSER DEFENSES

Children lack the same defenses to diseases that adults have. The immune system is not fully mature, the blood-brain barrier, which can block some toxicants, does not become fully effective until at least six months after birth, and enzymes that can detoxify substances can be undeveloped or underdeveloped in early life.

Children's blood proteins are less capable of binding to toxicants than are those of adults—leaving unbound toxicants to damage other tissues or organs—and their kidneys are slower to eliminate toxicants from their bodies than adults'.[200] Thus, greater vulnerability and lesser defenses substantially increase children's risks from any toxicants that tend to be in greater concentrations per body weight.

Two important organ systems—the brain and the immune system—are especially susceptible to diseases and dysfunction. The developing brain has windows of "unique susceptibility" because it must grow from a single cell into billions following "precise pathways" in the "correct sequence" to function properly. While considerable growth occurs in utero and in the first six months of life, brain development is not fully complete until adulthood.[201] The immune system is similarly sensitive; for both systems there seems to be "one chance to get it right."[202]

For reproductive systems there may or may not be only one chance to "get it right." However, Michael Skinner's research shows that it is comparatively easy to "get the reproductive system wrong," with very likely little chance to "make it right" later in life (examples illustrating this follow below).

It is easy to summarize the effects of toxicants on children. They are more susceptible to toxicants as their organs rapidly develop, and they have greater exposures per body weight. They have lesser defenses to resist diseases that may be triggered by exposures. They have a longer lifespan for diseases to develop than would a mature adult. If a child is exposed to pesticides that might trigger Parkinson's disease, the disease will likely appear much earlier in life than Parkinson's caused by middle-age pesticide exposure. Several adverse effects that appear in some organs seem irreversible—for the brain, the immune system, and likely the reproductive system.

Genetic variation can increase the susceptibility of children and adults alike. Some children are more susceptible to polycyclic aromatic hydrocarbons, typical byproducts of combustion.[203] Genetic variation makes others more vulnerable to the toxic effects of organophosphate pesticides.[204] Finally, some people, including children, are genetically more susceptible to the toxic effects of methylmercury.[205] No doubt other genetic susceptibilities will be uncovered, but these are currently known.

Moreover, some classes of substances, such as dioxin-like molecules, attach to the same receptor in a cell. When this occurs, the toxic effects add together, even if they are different substances, but appropriately they resemble dioxins.[206]

Similar phenomena can occur but by means of somewhat different mechanisms. Certain substances can affect different "upstream" pathways, producing jointly additive effects but not affecting the same cellular receptors. For example, dioxin-like PCBs (PCBs that resemble dioxins), non-dioxin-like PCBs, perchlorate (a component in rocket fuel and fireworks), and PBDEs, each traveling by a different biological pathway, can jointly reduce thyroid concentrations in people. This is especially important for pregnant women because thyroid concentrations that become too low during pregnancy can adversely affect a child's neurological development.[207] Similar generalized, independent additive effects disturb a developing immune system.[208]

The examples in the previous two paragraphs remind us that, while ordinarily the toxicity of products is assessed one at a time, people are exposed to multiple toxicants in their bodies. These might well and in some cases clearly do interact. Yet combinations of chemical creations are rarely studied for their joint effects. These could easily be worse than the toxicity of a sincle substance.

TOXICANT-INDUCED DISEASES OCCUR AT DIFFERENT DEVELOPMENTAL STAGES

Developmentally caused adverse effects can be manifested in different ways. Some diseases or dysfunctions result in obvious physical abnormalities, while some are less obvious, subtler, and more difficult to discern. Some may be neurological shortcomings that are revealed only after considerable testing. Others appear immediately after birth, while yet others may be long delayed, some possibly for many decades.

First trimester exposure to thalidomide, a pharmaceutical poorly tested for its toxicity, caused children to be born with obvious "seal limbs," shortened arms or legs, or misplaced appendages. Some other physical abnormalities would also have been seen immediately, such as deformed spines and missing ears or eyeballs. Other effects were subtler and took considerable testing to reveal, including neurological problems, heart disease, kidney abnormalities, and autism.[209] Valproic acid, ethanol (the active ingredient in alcohol), and misoprostol (used to prevent gastric ulcers) seem to trigger autism when an embryo is just beginning to develop (during embryogenesis).[210]

Pregnant women who have higher concentrations of phthalates in their bodies have elevated risks of giving birth to boys with a shortened anogenital distance, the distance between the anus and the penis.[211] These features would be evident at or shortly after birth. Typically, females have a shorter distance between the anus and the vagina than males do between the anus and penis. However, when males exhibit this, it suggests that their masculinization is truncated.

In animal studies, males dosed with phthalates retain nipples, like females. Human studies show that boys developing in utero in mothers with higher concentrations of phthalates may not be fully masculine; they are somewhat "feminized." These effects are especially worrisome because of the ubiquity of phthalates. Phthalates are endocrine disrupters that are present in toys, food packaging, pharmaceuticals, cosmetics, and personal-care products, among others.

Some toxin-caused neurological effects may be present at birth but not be identified until later, when functional abnormalities begin to appear.[212] Importantly, neurotoxicants can cause brain damage in developing children at much-lower concentrations than they do in adults. Various untested neurotoxicants (it is now known) have led to a variety of disorders. Lead in gasoline, paints, ceramic glazes, and numerous other products can contribute to neurological deficits in concentration, memory, and cognition; they also promote disruptive behavior from poor impulse control.[213] In utero exposure to methylmercury from mothers eating fish contaminated with the substance resulted in cerebral palsy and sometimes limb abnormalities (obvious conditions at birth). Methylmercury also caused sensory disturbance, poor muscle control, mental retardation, and a constricted visual field.[214] Arsenic, PCBs, various solvents, manganese, and numerous pesticides (not well tested for neurotoxicity at least initially) can also contribute to neurological disorders.

Some childhood cancers begin in utero but do not appear until a few years after birth. Acute lymphoblastic leukemia (ALL) and acute myeloid childhood leukemia (AML) seem to be triggered by a chromosomal translocation in utero (a first hit) typically followed by a major immunological event after birth (a second hit), which together trigger the cancers. Exogenous or endogenous in utero exposures can cause the first hit.[215] Exposures to pesticides are associated with ALL (relative risk of 11:1) and with AML (relative risk of 14:1), while exposures to paints and pigments, metal dusts, and sawdust also seem to elevate risks.[216]

Diethylstilbestrol (DES), a poorly tested pharmaceutical approved for use in 1947,[217] initiated the first stage of disease in utero in female offspring, but its effects did not clinically appear until the women turned about 20 years old, when they contracted vaginal/cervical cancer. Females exposed to DES in utero were 40 times more likely to develop vaginal/cervical cancers than children not so exposed. After age 40 the same daughters "have approximately twice the risk of breast cancer as unexposed women of the same age and with similar risk factors."[218] There are later associated fertility problems such as premature delivery, stillbirth (relative risk 2.45:1), neonatal death (relative risk 8.12:1), miscarriage during the second trimester (relative risk 3.77:1), and infertility (relative risk 2.37:1).[219] DES sons may be at some biological risks, but they do appear to have greater psychopathology than in men not exposed to DES.[220] There is some suggestive evidence that "DES granddaughters and DES grandsons may have a slightly higher risk of cancer and birth defects, including hypospadias [misplaced urethra] in DES grandsons."[221] Many of these latter problems were revealed only after decades of research and any concomitant misery experienced by those with the diseases and by their families.

During the teenage years, toxic exposures can trigger diseases that have higher risks than adults with the same exposures. Teenage women with DDT exposures around the time of puberty contracted breast cancer 20 years later at rates five times higher than adult women with comparable exposures.[222] Women born to mothers who had substantial exposures to DDT half a century ago are now contracting breast cancer at rates four times higher than women not exposed to DDT in utero. This is a second-generation effect with possible alternative explanations ruled out.[223] Radiation similarly "increases breast cancer risk most strongly when exposures occur early in life."[224] Importantly, women seem to have particularly critical periods when they are more susceptible to having breast cancer triggered: "during fetal life, adolescence, and early reproductive life, particularly before the first full-term pregnancy."[225]

An utterly fascinating study not involving toxic chemicals in Sweden found that overeating by teenage boys just prior to puberty seems to increase risks for cardiovascular disease and diabetes in their grandsons. I include it as an example of an effect occurring during teenage years that has consequences not for the individual involved or for that boy's children, but for his grandchildren. The researchers suggest that a "nutrition-linked mechanism through the male line" explains diseases that can be initiated during development but not be manifested until a later generation.[226]

During development, the immune system goes through several functional changes that make people (and other mammals) vulnerable to toxic exposures. As a result, toxic exposures that might predict immune system dysfunction in adults do not adequately predict immune dysfunctions that can occur from childhood exposures—children are much more sensitive.[227] In addition, various significant childhood diseases—asthma, type 1 diabetes, inflammatory bowel disease, respiratory infections/rhinitis, recurrent otitis media, pediatric celiac, juvenile arthritis, and Kawasaki disease—that result from immune system dysfunction are "associated with increased risk of several secondary conditions, many of which appear only later in life."[228] Some of these childhood diseases are caused by toxicants, such as PCBs, dioxin, and tobacco smoke (which contains heavy metals, benzene, and polycyclic aromatic hydrocarbons). Infant animal exposure to immunotoxicants shows there can be greater dose sensitivity, severity of effects, and persistence along with a wider and different range of effects than adult exposures.[229]

The above shows that early-life exposures with disease consequences are not the end of the story. In a double whammy, primary immune system dysfunctions can exhibit unified susceptibility patterns later in life. Scientists seem to "know far less about the immunological safety of chemicals and drugs for these sensitive sub-populations than for adults."[230] Thus, we need to identify toxicants that can adversely affect the immune system, since early-life dysfunctions seem to be irreversible and can then lead to a lifetime of health problems. Since the 1976 TSCA does not require toxicity data, these adverse effects are almost certainly unknown in new chemicals under that law or in products that have been grandfathered as safe.

EXQUISITE SENSITIVITY: TINY DOSES CAN POSE PROBLEMS

Serious health problems in children can be initiated during different periods of development, in part because of their extreme sensitivity to toxicants. As already noted, the same concentration of DDT elevates the risk of breast cancer in teenagers compared with adults. However, for some substances, quite tiny and fleeting doses may be sufficient to trigger diseases.

A single dose of one 50-milligram (mg) or 100 mg pill caused malformations in at least one thalidomide baby. The mother did not have to take large or continual doses to trigger seal limbs in her child; one ill-timed pill was sufficient.[231] Similarly, animal studies have found that a single dose of valproic acid, an anti-epileptic drug, early in embryonic life can cause autism-like behavior.[232]

Some substances are not so discriminating in causing adverse effects during development. There appears to be no threshold for lead or mutagenic carcinogens for toxicity during development, early childhood, or even adulthood.[233] A single dose of DES (and some other synthetic estrogens) is sufficient to cause obesity in mice.[234]

Often, hormones can have toxic effects at quite low doses, causing greater harm than larger doses. High doses of tamoxifen inhibit breast cancer growth, lower concentrations stimulate breast cancer cell growth, and the highest doses are acutely toxic. Endocrine-disrupting chemicals can have unfortunate effects at low doses that would not be predicted by testing responses at higher doses. Hormonal reactions contradict the received view that the "dose makes the poison." Moreover, low-dose effects seem to be "remarkably common in studies of natural hormones and [endocrine-disrupting chemicals]."[235]

Often, children experience worse effects than adults at the same dose. Thalidomide did not cause any lasting damage to women who took it during pregnancy, but some of them gave birth to children with a wide range of birth defects. DES mothers did not contract cervical cancer, as did some of their daughters. However, later in life the mothers were at higher risk for breast cancer than women who did not take DES. Their daughters often suffered the double whammy of cervical/vaginal cancer at about the age of 20 and then later breast cancer.

THE TIMING OF EXPOSURES AND TRANSGENERATIONAL EFFECTS

Recent animal data exploring multigenerational effects of toxic exposures show that exposing germ cells in utero to toxicants can contribute to serious diseases that are multigenerational (spanning more than one generation) or even transgenerational (spanning generations out to great-grandchildren or great- great-grandchildren).

Pregnant rats exposed to an individual pesticide or a dose of BPA when reproductive organs are developing in male fetuses can cause sperm damage, sterility, and a host of cancers when the males become adults (first generation) and in their sons' offspring (second generation) after being bred with wild types of females. Subsequent generations showed a wider range of diseases: prostate disease, kidney disease, immune system abnormalities, testis abnormalities, and tumor development. Thus, a brief period of exposure in a pregnant rat can affect family lines for an indefinite period.[236] These studies suggest concerns for humans.

Similar experiments with a range of substances revealed somewhat analogous effects in female offspring. Professor Michael Skinner exposed pregnant rats to one of the following compounds—(1) vinclozolin, a pesticide, (2) a combination of the pesticides permethrin and DEET (N,N-Diethyl-*meta*-toluamide), (3) a plastics mixture, (4) dioxin, or (5) jet fuel—during gestation, when female reproductive organs develop (days 8–15). The subsequent four generations of female offspring developed polycystic ovarian disease and primary ovarian insufficiency (POI). Polycystic ovarian disease consists of infrequent ovulation, high androgen levels, multiple persistent ovarian cysts, and often related insulin resistance. These effects, demonstrated in rats, are seen in 6–18% of women; thus, if chemical exposures caused similar effects in human populations, they would be quite significant and disturbing. POI is the name for a decreased primordial follicle pool of eggs, the precursors of fully developed eggs. When this pool is smaller, it tends to reduce the chances of pregnancy over a lifetime. Again, these results were demonstrated in rats, but in humans POI appears in about 1% of women.[237]

Skinner's lab has also found that in utero exposure to DDT at concentrations seen in humans can transgenerationally promote obesity in experimental animals across four generations. Diseases in offspring associated with a one-time exposure include heritable germ line epimutations, testis disease, polycystic ovarian disease, immune abnormalities, kidney disease, and some tumors.[238]

In the 1950s–1960s, US citizens had 100% DDT exposure. In my hometown, trucks drove up and down streets spraying DDT on trees and lawns to kill mosquitoes. My parents used DDT in a hand sprayer to kill them in the house. At that time, about 5% of the population was obese. Today, two or three generations later, the obesity rate in the United States is 40%. While obesity has many causes, Skinner's animal experiments suggest that DDT may predispose mammals to obesity later in life and that the effects can be transgenerational. Early-life DDT exposure may contribute to the current "epidemic of obesity."[239]

Most of the examples described above reference exposures occurring in utero. However, what about fathers? They too can contribute to adverse effects in children. These have been called "bad daddy" factors. When men are exposed to Paxil, anesthetic gases, morphine, lead, mercury, pesticides, solvents, dyes, and paints, this can increase risks of miscarriages or other prenatal or neonatal problems.[240] A father's nutrition or stress can also affect the health of his future children. What men need "to know is that [their] life experience leaves biological traces on [their] children."[241]

Thus, both contaminated men and women could contribute to their children's diseases or dysfunctions. This is important for occupational exposures. If either parent is contaminated with a toxicant at the wrong time, it could affect the future health of their children. Workplaces can lead to these problems, despite early congressional passage of the Occupational Safety and Health Act (1970), which aimed to protect employees from toxicants. This argues for much more stringent occupational standards for adults to prevent some diseases in their future children.

TRANSIENT CHEMICAL EXPOSURES CAN BECOME BIOLOGICALLY EMBEDDED

The upshot of the above is that what appear to be *transient, tiny, but often ill-timed* exposures can become *biologically embedded* in individuals, in their children or grandchildren (multigenerational), and, with appropriate timing, in family lines (transgenerational). Sometimes even brief, one-time, or even fairly short-term exposures can become entrenched biologically. This in turn can cause diseases or dysfunctions in the affected animal or human offspring, or in later generations.

The evidentiary picture for the developmental basis of disease is something like a pointillist painting: parts of the picture filled with numerous data points, others partially filled, some blank, but the general background reasonably solid. There is substantial scientific evidence that our children are among the most vulnerable of citizens, they are highly permeable to chemical invasions, and some in fact are being harmed. We also know that portions of the population are at live risk on the basis of findings in animal data.

LEGAL FAILURES

Children, quite susceptible to toxic substances from embryonic life through to adulthood, are poorly protected under postmarket laws.

Because of legislative choices, most substances have minimal or no data that scientists can use to protect the public. Consequently, public health agencies and impartial scientists cannot quickly reduce exposures or eliminate risks, due to the pace of scientific studies. Fierce opposition from companies keeps their products in commerce even longer, extending risks and any diseases they cause. Citizens, children and adults alike, have been harmed because of legal shortcomings. Current laws, as well as how science is used to try to protect our most-susceptible citizens, fail to do the job. Accurate scientific tools could be used to protect citizens earlier in the lives of products, but apart from pharmaceuticals and pesticides, until the 1976 TSCA was amended by the Lautenberg Act they had not been. Going forward they will be, although exposures to substances of unknown toxicity will continue for some time even with the amendments (more in Chapter 4).

In other areas of our lives we do not treat fellow community members as postmarket laws do. Pharmaceutical and pesticide laws, along with the ethics of medical testing, stand in marked contrast. Pharmaceutical laws require extensive testing in order to determine both beneficial effects from a drug as well as any risky side effects. Pesticide laws are somewhat similar, seeking to determine the efficacy of substances for eradicating insects, fungi, or rodents, inter alia, while ensuring there is a reasonable certainty of no harm to humans. In addition, medical experiments on people who, for example, would be given experimental pharmaceuticals or various forms of therapy (e.g., gene therapy) require prudent measures to ensure their safety. There must be sufficient preparation and prior testing to identify potentials risks to participants *before* they participate in the experiment; concern for the participant is central, and typically children may not be experimental subjects. Moreover, such tests must have some independent and impartial review both of the scientific soundness of the experiment and its ethical acceptability.[242]

Of course, not every drug, pesticide, or medical experiment poses risks. Some exposures may have no risks at all. However, these laws and the ethics of medical research require *prudent and sensible testing* for possible risks to those exposed because they could be exposed to *possible* risks.

In these three areas there is a quite different conception of the relations between citizens who create chemicals and those who are exposed to (or taking) them, and how science is used to protect them (or not) from potential risks compared with postmarket laws. However, the problems with postmarket laws are deeper, revealing how citizens are treated unjustly in several different ways.

INJUSTICES

If we combine the facts about children's vulnerability and how they have been harmed under postmarket laws together with a well-known theory of justice, it becomes clear that postmarket laws and chemical creations from companies treat numerous citizens unjustly. Several features of John Rawls's theory of justice provide the resources for this assessment.

Theories of distributive justice, of which his is a prominent example, quintessentially concern relations between people—how should they be treated vis-à-vis one another in the community. What constitutes just treatment of fellow members of the community? Rawls focuses on how "basic institutions" in a community are designed and administered in governing relations between people. These include the law, along with economic, political, and educational institutions. I extend his idea to public health institutions authorized by law.

One component of justice is Rawls's first principle: each person should "have an equal right to the most extensive liberty compatible with a like liberty for all."[243] The broad and important fundamental rights incorporated into this principle provide equal foundations and zones of protection for all in the community. They protect citizens so they may develop their life plans, by congregating with others to pursue them if they wish, pursuing religious or comprehensive philosophical views, participating in and influencing political institutions that govern their lives, being treated equally under the rule of law, and being free from physical invasions of their integrity and psychological oppression. This last right he calls "freedom of the person," which is important for our purposes.

The freedom of the person seeks to ensure that people in the community are "free from psychological oppression and physical assault and dismemberment ([constituting] integrity of the person)."[244] Freedom from physical invasion and psychological oppression and having a secure sense of one's integrity as a person are major prerequisites to many other activities and carrying out life plans.

Harms: When the products or activities of others *harm* a fellow citizen, this is an obvious violation of one's freedom. Some harms might be mild and short term, while others could be more serious and last a lifetime, with various possibilities in between. The range of possible harms would be injustices under the equal liberties principle.

Exposure to trichloroethylene (TCE) with accompanying diseases illustrates several different kinds and degrees of injustices. TCE was first produced in 1925 and was sometimes used as an ingredient in foods and cosmetics before it was banned for those uses in 1977, but mainly it had industrial applications.[245] When TCE was introduced and likely for many years after that, if the law and public health institutions permitted citizens to be exposed to it, not knowing whether it was toxic or not, this posed a subtle injustice, to which I will return later in this chapter.

More noticeably, TCE causes minor and major harms. Short-term exposures can cause drowsiness, mucous membrane irritation, confusion, and headaches. Slightly longer exposures can have affect perception, memory, reaction time, and dexterity. These appear to be comparatively minor harms and injustices that ordinarily would resolve in reasonably short order.

Longer exposures—one month to 15 years—might cause short-term memory loss, sleep disturbances, vertigo, and even difficulty in controlling one's muscles (ataxia).[246] These more-serious harms are also first-principle injustices, but not even the most serious.

Because TCE poses risks to the central nervous system, the endocrine (hormonal) system, and the immune system in adults, these can lead to more serious long-term effects. If pregnant women are exposed, TCE can cause risk of miscarriage, along with neural-tube or cardiac defects, and childhood cancer.[247] It is carcinogenic to humans[248] and causes Parkinson's disease.[249]

If TCE exposure causes more-significant biological problems in children, along with cancer, Parkinson's disease, or other long-term neurological problems in adults, which it does, these too are unjust, but much more serious. These problems are intrusive and long term and have substantial life-changing effects. When such diseases significantly interfere with a person's biological functioning sufficient to prevent pursuit of normal opportunities over a lifetime, this undermines the affected person's opportunity ranges.

Undermining fair equality of opportunity: A second major component of Rawls's theory of justice captures this thought—his conception of the fair-equality-of-opportunity principle (FEOP). Those who have the same level of talent, ability, and motivation to use them "should have the same prospect of success regardless of their initial place in the social system. In all sectors of society there should be roughly equal prospects of culture and achievement for everyone similarly motivated and endowed."[250] When these conditions obtain, citizens have fair equality of opportunity; when they do not, they are denied fair equality of opportunity.

This is conditional equality between persons: *if* two people have approximately *equal* talents, abilities, and motivations, they should have approximately equal chances of obtaining the same good things or goals in life, should they choose to pursue them. Rawls does not claim that every person regardless of abilities and motivations should have similar chances of becoming a doctor, lawyer, or federal judge.

Basic institutions in a community are strategically important in ensuring FEOP. For Rawls, education is a most important basic institution that helps ensure this, but not the only one as Norman Daniels has argued.

Serious diseases or dysfunctions (e.g., more-serious maladies caused by TCE exposures; see above) can constrain one's ability to be a normal, fully functioning person over a complete life from birth to death. If health maladies reduce one's opportunities to construct and revise life plans, or undermine them in substantial ways, this transgresses a broader idea of fair equality of opportunity.

Consequently, health protection and healthcare institutions are strategically important in securing fair equality of opportunity for people. For instance, serious diseases can cause long-term impairments, disrupt education, interrupt careers, and interfere with plans for different aspects of one's life at different stages. Chronic illnesses such as asthma can cause emergency room visits and burden activities that require good health. Some diseases can frustrate or eliminate choices in one's life. A person cannot choose later in life to climb Mt. Kilimanjaro if he or she has contracted a toxic-induced leukemia, as Brain Milward did.

When poor health occurs, fair equality of opportunity requires that there should be healthcare institutions in society that are equally available to all to cure or ameliorate diseases, to the extent that medical science can do so. If a community does not have such institutions or they are of poor quality for various classes of people in society, this would be unjust. Thus, Daniels argues that well-functioning healthcare and public health institutions are strategically important for ensuring just treatment of citizens. They should *minimize* the departures of persons from being normal, fully functioning persons over a complete life span and should *correct departures from normal healthy functioning* with medical and rehabilitative services, and for those who cannot be completely restored to normal functioning, just institutions should *maintain them* as close as possible to this goal over a complete life span.[251]

Daniels was largely concerned with diseases that "just happen to us," such as mumps, measles, polio, typhoid fever, scarlet fever, and so on. For these we typically would need access to healthcare and physicians. While he mentioned the need for environmental cleanliness and protections for workers, his discussion was limited.

I have extended his idea further and in more detail. Thus, if one group of citizens produces chemical creations of unknown toxicity that invade other citizens, and these other citizens then contract serious diseases, such as cancer, Parkinson's disease, or neurological disorders, the institutions that permit this and the companies who made the products, not knowing their toxicity, have violated citizens' equality of opportunity and are unjust.

Consequently, if people exposed to TCE contract less serious, nonpermanent maladies, this would be unjust under Rawls's freedom principle. In addition, if they were to contract more serious diseases from TCE (e.g., cancers or Parkinson's disease) that interfere with their normal biology and curtail their opportunity ranges, this would be a violation of both the freedom of the person and the fair opportunity principles. Similar points could be made about exposure to formaldehyde, discussed in the introduction.

Battery violations: There is also a less visible, subtler injustice under postmarket laws—most citizens are subject to moral and legal "battery" under the 1976 TSCA.

A legal battery occurs when an agent knowingly causes another person, "directly or indirectly, to come in contact with a foreign substance in a manner which the other will reasonably regard as offensive."[252] This "dignitary tort" protects a person's autonomy, and personal dignity, and, less directly, one's "health."[253] Actual physical harm need not occur; a "technical invasion of the integrity of the plaintiff's person by even an entirely harmless, but offensive, contact entitles him to vindication of his legal right by an award of nominal damages, and the establishment of the tort cause of action entitles him also to compensation for the mental disturbance inflicted upon him."[254]

To establish battery, a plaintiff must show "that the defendant committed a voluntary act with the intent to cause a wrongful contact and the contact occurred."[255] Spitting in someone's face, daubing filth [excrement] on a towel a person is likely to use, forcibly removing a hat, putting offensive ingredients in food, setting out poisoned food for someone to eat, or delivering an unappreciated kiss all constitute battery.[256]

Originally, battery gave invaded persons legal recourse for offensive violations instead of their resorting to the self-help of violence (that would breach the criminal law) in an effort to receive satisfaction for indignities. It is socially quite useful and important to have a legal cause of action for which one could receive some redress after being spit on, instead of responding with physical violence. Battery presupposes that citizens have certain social boundaries that protect bodily integrity and individual autonomy in order to create and secure essential status relations between persons and to provide space for social interactions.[257]

A federal district court amplified the idea: "Underlying this theory of liability is, of course, the general feeling that a person of sound mind has a right to determine, even as against his physician, what is to be done to his body."[258] "[O]ther persons do not have the right to interfere with the person of another unless he or she validly consents to such an interference."[259] Consent negates the claim of battery.[260]

A clear example of battery occurred from exposure to DES in the 1960s and 1970s. Some physicians at the time believed that DES might help prevent miscarriages, but they were unaware of risks to female fetuses. In 1978 Patsy Mink and other pregnant women became unknown subjects in a DES experiment as part of their prenatal care. They did not know they were given DES and did not even know they were part of an experiment.

When they discovered how the University of Chicago had treated them, they brought a lawsuit in battery (among other causes of action). The court endorsed their battery cause of action, ruling that the instigator need not act with a "desire or purpose to bring about physical results"; it is enough if the "actor believes [the consequences] *are substantially certain* to follow" from the action (emphasis added).[261]

Battery from invasions of untested industrial chemicals: The wrong of battery captures in major part what is amiss when manufacturers create chemical products, being substantially certain that they will invade others' bodies, and do little or nothing to determine any risks they might pose to fellow citizens. As the legal scholar Mary Lyndon notes, "If it is tortious to seriously insult or startle someone, it would seem an even greater transgression of social boundaries to inflict a silent, invisible bodily contact with a possible toxicant, leaving those 'touched' to wait whatever may come. The common law invokes the actual lived experience of toxic exposure as a source of governance, adding substance to the flat numerical risk estimates that regulatory experts produce."[262]

Exposures to TCE or formaldehyde or C8 illustrate this. If people were exposed to any of these, none initially tested for its toxicity, they suffered legal battery and were treated unjustly under the freedom of the person principle. Silent, invisible substances that were possibly toxic (all are now well-known toxicants) transgressed their social boundaries, leaving them "'touched' to wait whatever may come." Bodily invasions of untested substances constitute violations of a person's integrity (an aspect of freedom of the person) just as surely as spitting in someone's face or daubing filth on a towel a person might use.

Consequently, as I argued elsewhere, "Combining the different elements, if [a chemical manufacturer] is *substantially certain* that his act will cause foreign substances to *come in contact* with another person without consent and in a manner that the recipient would *reasonably regard as offensive* even if at the time the person is unaware of the contact, the agent has committed battery."[263]

Lyndon, in an extensive discussion of battery, concurs. "In battery law, the test for offensiveness is a community standard. The Restatement (Second) of Torts holds that a bodily contact is offensive 'if it offends a reasonable sense of personal dignity' and is 'one which would offend the ordinary person.'"[264] The invading substance may or may not be toxic and the person may or may not suffer illness or harm. The injustice consists of simply being invaded by substances of unknown toxicity, but then having to wait to see if any physical harm occurs.[265]

Cognitive dissonance: We have seen earlier how under the laws for pharmaceuticals and pesticides and under the principles guiding medical experiments collectively we place high priority on using science to test substances and understand potential risks *before people are exposed.* The rules in these different circumstances require *prudent testing* for possible risks to those exposed. The principles guiding these areas of our lives also reveal quite different conceptions of the relations between people and how scientific studies could be used to protect us from risks compared with living under postmarket laws. This should create cognitive dissonance between life under postmarket laws and under premarket laws (and principles for medical experiments).

Under postmarket laws there are no legally required toxicity tests prior to exposures, no preparations, and no reasonable assurances of safety. There are no careful assessments of safe exposures. There are no special safeguards for children, and the health and welfare of citizens are not of central concern. There are no commitments to use science to identify adverse effects until well after exposures have occurred and there is evidence of risks or harms. There is nothing like independent scientific or ethical oversight to ensure protections for the populace. (Under the 2016 Lautenberg Act if the EPA does its job well, these problems should be better addressed.)

Diseases can adversely affect distributions of income and wealth: As a fourth, but less certain point about injustice, toxicant-induced diseases sometimes affect the distribution of income and wealth in a community and sometimes can unjustly skew income distributions.

If diseases cause substantial decrements in wealth because of medical costs, reduced ability to work, or loss of jobs altogether, these would be *externalities* imposed on the affected people. They would be unjust cost impositions. Negative externalities are social costs of an activity imposed on others that are not incorporated into the costs of the activity or associated products. If I pollute the river, dump trash on the courthouse lawn, or expose the community to lead, I have imposed costs on the community, instead of reducing the pollution, paying to take trash to the community dump, or more carefully controlling the lead. Similarly, if a company exposes employees to toxicants that cause them diseases, as DuPont and others have, instead of installing safety devices that could have prevented them, it has imposed negative externalities on them.

Ken Wamsley, whom we met in the introduction, had to declare bankruptcy because of his C8-caused ulcerative colitis and subsequent colon cancer. Such costs may also and often do exacerbate unequal distributions of income and wealth. This would be a fourth dimension of Rawlsian injustice under his "difference principle." If exposures to toxicants were to cause decreases in income and wealth, this would affect the distribution of income and wealth and exacerbate economic maldistributions, this would be unjust.[266]

Lower socioeconomic groups are likely to live in contaminated neighborhoods or racially segregated areas that also tend to be contaminated, to work in jobs with more-toxic exposures, to drink contaminated water (as in Flint, Michigan), or to live in houses contaminated with deteriorating lead point.[267] As a consequence they are likely to have more diseases and dysfunctions than citizens who live in "cleaner" communities. Coping with such diseases is likely to reduce their income and wealth. In short, they experience "externalities" from others' activities.[268]

Toxic chemical creations might cause a wide range of negative disease externalities—retarded or impaired mental development, decreased IQ, poor memory, antisocial behavior, or other neurological deficiencies; vaginal cancer at age 20; breast, prostate, kidney, or bone cancers; or early parkinsonism—many of which could have been prevented with adequate toxicity testing before commercialization.

THE INJUSTICE OF POSTMARKET LAWS

The strands of this chapter lead to some preliminary conclusions. Children are among the most vulnerable of our citizenry and at greater risk from chemical creations because of their biology and the diseases that can originate during their developmental stages. In addition, because they have a longer lifetime for diseases to develop, this adds to the urgency to protect them.

However, postmarket laws, including the 1976 TSCA, permit companies to create chemical products that in fact put children at risk, but no one may know it. (The 2016 Lautenberg Act should reduce these problems for new products if it is implemented well.) Such laws simply cannot prevent diseases induced by toxic substances during development, because protections come too late. (The amended TSCA will at best quite sluggishly reduce these risks (Chapter 4).) Moreover, even when conscientious, impartial scientists seek to develop good data showing risks or harm, there can be frustrating delays in reducing or removing the risks because studies move at their own pace. Inadequately funded and understaffed public health institutions, obfuscating actions by affected companies, and less honorable intransigence aggravate the problems.

Children and adults alike are treated unjustly by battery from invasion by untested substances, moderate harms, and opportunity-truncating diseases and dysfunctions. Indeed, many children have been condemned to the last fate because they suffer from lead poisoning, childhood cancer, serious asthma, intellectual disability, autism, attention deficit disorder, and childhood cancers attributable to chemical exposures. The healthcare costs attributable to these exposures were estimated to be $76.6 billion in 2008. I put this in greater context in chapter 4.[269] The outcomes are also tragic—when people are harmed, depending on the seriousness of disease, they likely experience greater or lesser misery and suffering.

What is the solution? In brief, we should require premarket testing of products somewhat similar but not identical to premarket testing of pharmaceuticals and pesticides. I have suggested this elsewhere and say more about it in chapter 4.[270] However, general chemical creations can be biologically active and harm humans and the environment, as the Council on Environmental Quality understood in 1971, only now the effects are more widespread. Thus, these products should be tested for their toxicity before they enter commerce, the environment, and our bodies. The tests would not need to be as extensive as they are for pharmaceuticals because there is no reason to test for a therapeutic (beneficial) dose of each substance. Neither would they need to be tested as fully as pesticides because they do not have to have beneficial biological effects, as do pesticides. Instead, general chemicals need only be reviewed for various toxic endpoints to avoid the kinds of problems that were caused by children's and adult's exposures to known products. These recommendations have good company—they are supported by three National Academy of Sciences committees (more in chapter 4).[271] By enacting the Lautenberg Act Congress has now concurred.

The European Union (EU) has realized these issues, adopting improved testing for approximately 30,000 new and existing chemicals. The law, compiling and strengthening existing legislation, is known by the acronym REACH—the Registration, Evaluation, Authorisation and Restriction of Chemicals. REACH requires specified data on each substance that is manufactured, used, or distributed in Europe.[272]

The practical import of REACH is summarized in the epigram "No data, no market."[273] If no toxicity tests have been conducted on a product, a new chemical may not enter the market and an existing one may not continue in commerce. Companies must be licensed by the EU to manufacture, sell, or distribute the product in the EU, but licensing is conditional upon companies doing appropriate testing and ensuring their safety to an appropriate EU agency.[274] Tests must provide reasonable assurance to the EU of no significant risks from toxicants.[275]

The legislation "is based on the principle that responsibility for testing and ensuring the safety of the products rests with those who manufacture, import, place on the market or use these substances." They must ensure that the substances do not adversely affect human health or the environment.[276] The same testing protocols apply both to new and existing chemicals, eliminating previous asymmetries between them.

A product's tonnage, a surrogate for citizens' exposures, guides the kinds and extensiveness of tests to which it would be subject, beginning at 1 ton per year. Escalating numbers and the intensiveness of tests increase as production grows.[277] The ultimate aim of the legislation is to replace more dangerous products with less dangerous ones when where there are appropriate alternatives. This will make the market for chemical creations safer to the public over time.

REACH seeks to broadly screen thousands of substances, but there are some concerns about it. Pursuit of breadth under REACH could sacrifice some depth of analysis because it could leave some risks undetected.[278] However, the total costs of testing likely preclude both in-depth analysis and broad coverage of each product. REACH partially remedies this by permitting greater testing "to be triggered on the basis of initial results."[279] Perhaps more worrisome is that protocols under REACH may not require tests for some "relevant end points and life stages," such as fetuses, children, and the very old. Nonetheless, REACH protocols are an improvement compared to 1976 TSCA and other US postmarket laws.[280]

REACH no doubt raises concern about the costs of testing 30,000 chemical products. However, a closer look suggests that testing this universe of substances would be far less daunting than one might suppose (chapter 4).

REACH conditions access to markets on the basis of identifying and reducing risks from products. This creates a substantially different moral and legal relationship between citizens in a country and firms seeking to do business within it. In contrast, under the 1976 TSCA and other postmarket laws, companies in effect have a legal right to market products unless and until the products show that they cause unreasonable risks of harm. The public had to bear the consequences. Under the Lautenberg Act this will improve for proposed *new chemical products*. The thousands of substances already in commerce will remain there, putting the public at risk until they are assessed and exposures reduced if need be.

CONCLUSION

In an earlier era, public health officials sought to prevent diseases and dysfunctions by chlorinating drinking water, cleaning up sewage, and discovering vaccines to immunize people against diseases before they occurred. Those maladies have largely disappeared from community life, at least in developed countries. However, analogous solutions are not available for any of the diseases caused by toxic exposures during development; they result from the products created by our fellow citizens—the chemical manufacturers—and have been legally permitted. There are also no vaccines to protect the public from lead, phthalates, bisphenol A, formaldehyde, TCE, PBDEs, or C8.

To reduce and to go a long way toward eliminating many of the diseases discussed in this chapter, as well as any associated personal tragedies, we should choose legal and institutional changes to screen out toxicants as best as we can before the public and employees are exposed. Such actions bear some analogy to cleansing water supplies and cleaning up animal waste and sewage, only now we would be cleaning up our chemical exposures, which we could regard as wastes, by separating nontoxic (or vastly less toxic) chemicals from more toxic products.

With the Lautenberg Act Congress has now modified when the EPA should use science in the service of public health for new products. It has recognized that scientific tools can be better used to protect us with premarket toxicity testing laws and seeks to regularize and speed up review of existing substances. This will better serve justice in the community. And, there also appears to be considerable monetary benefits in doing so (Chapter 4).

Premarket testing of *new substances* will go some way toward preventing childhood cancers, brain dysfunctions, and the feminization of boys. It may also reduce some women's breast cancer and various reproductive harms. Molecular contamination is inevitable, unavoidable because of who we are as a species, and how permeable we are; there are no places to hide. Existing chemical products pose a different problem (Chapter 4).

Moving toward better protections from general chemicals will require community support for public health agencies to do their jobs well and political pressure to create more just institutions and a safer community in which to live. While I do not want to be a Pollyanna on this issue, some of these pressures probably led to the Lautenberg amendments, but there remains more to do (Chapter 4).

Chapter 3

How Do Obscure Supreme Court Decisions Affect Me?

INTRODUCTION

When public health laws fail to protect citizens from hazardous chemical creations (or other products or activities), the tort or personal-injury law is the branch of the legal system that offers the possibility of redressing their injuries. However, because of molecules' tiny size and the difficulties of tracing their causal paths, scientific expertise and studies are also needed in the tort law. Decisions by the US Supreme Court since the mid-1990s have introduced substantial changes in how science is used in the law. The law-science relationship has been modified in three Supreme Court cases that address the testimony of scientific experts in the law, the so-called Daubert trilogy: *Daubert v. Merrell Dow Pharmaceuticals* (1993), *General Electric v. Joiner* (1997), and *Kumho Tire v. Carmichael* (1999).[281] These decisions gave trial and appellate judges increased responsibilities to review the science pertinent to legal decisions.

Supreme Court decisions by themselves may seem remote, arcane, and difficult to interpret. When they involve decisions concerning science—a topic most find even more esoteric—this compounds the difficulties, perhaps exponentially. Consequently, the decisions that changed the law may be difficult to appreciate because they occurred behind something of a "science veil."[282]

Giving judges greater duties to consider the science needed for a legal determination required that they increase their scientific sophistication and, to some extent, this occurred. However, they still need to refine their understanding. The esoteric nature of science and scientific reasoning is problematic, but not just for ordinary people. Judges have also struggled to properly appreciate different kinds of studies and their pertinence for legal decisions.

Nonetheless, judicial decisions in the tort law can have major impacts on our lives and the communities in which we live. Some courts have mistakenly understood and applied scientific studies. Mistaken decisions reduce injured parties' possibilities of just redress for injuries caused by others. Judicial errors also send misleading signals about how safe products are and should be; in more technical language, they can reduce the deterrent effects of the tort law. Errors can also disadvantage defendants if their science or experts are excluded.

While unfortunate outcomes for some injured parties have been one consequence of these legal changes, the recent decision in the U.S. Court of Appeals for the First Circuit involving Brian Milward (followed by numerous other courts) signals better interpretations of the Supreme Court cases, excellent understanding of science and scientific reasoning, improvements for compensatory justice, and, potentially, the promise of a somewhat safer world to live in.

THE TORT LAW

The tort law is the major area of law that permits a person who believes he or she has been injured by the actions or products of others to "put matters right." This would occur by requiring "the harm-doer to restore something to the person harmed, or to repair a damaged object, or (when the unharmed position cannot be restored, as it usually cannot be) to compensate the harm sufferer."[283]

In order to do this, the injured party, the plaintiff, must show that a defendant (or the defendants) breached the law, that the plaintiff suffered an injury recognized as compensable by the law, and that the defendant's breach caused and was the proximate cause of the plaintiff's injuries. All these elements of a tort offense must be established by a preponderance of the evidence—showing that the elements are more likely than not true to the satisfaction of a jury. If a plaintiff succeeds in these showings, she would receive some rectification for the harm she suffered. If she does not satisfy each of these elements, she will not receive redress.

The tort law also has some future deterrent effects—general deterrence, deterrence by example, and deterrence by reform—although how effective they are is not clear. The threat of possible tort lawsuits for risky behavior or products creates *general deterrence*, discouraging some unsafe behavior. No one likes to be sued; it is costly, time consuming, and a likely source of personal anxiety. In addition, seeing others lose a tort suit can *set an example* and deter others from similar potentially harmful activities or products. Finally, if a defendant loses a tort suit, this may lead to *reform* of activities, products, or behavior that led to the legal defeat. Conversely, if plaintiffs lose, this sends a message that the activity or product was not as unjurious as claimed.

The tort law importantly backs up other legal failures. As we discussed in chapter 2, more than 300 man-made substances contaminate US citizens, and there is good evidence that many of these are causing harm because postmarket laws and sometimes premarket laws fail to protect the public. Consequently, any deterrent effects of the tort law could help make the world a somewhat safer place from risky activities and products. We can see this by the tort law's effects on providing compensation for children harmed by exposures to lead, a quite harmful substance (chapter 2).

Children's lead exposure can cause a variety of neurological problems, such as "lower IQs, violent behavior, motor skill problems and attention disorders [ADHD]" and later in life cardiovascular disease.[284] It is surprisingly pernicious; researchers can find no safe level during development, in early childhood, or even in adulthood.[285]

Recently, there have been some successes in the tort law in redressing some injuries from lead when public health and other laws failed citizens. In one legal case, plaintiffs and defendants reached a settlement for seven children who had been exposed to a lead-mining site and contracted various neurological problems as a result.[286] In an unrelated tort case, plaintiffs won $358 million in compensatory and punitive damages for injuries to 16 children exposed to airborne lead from a local smelter.[287]

These children were not "protected," however—they were harmed, likely with lifelong disease consequences. They and their families received compensation for their injuries and medical costs, inter alia. Even though compensation to some extent makes life easier for injured parties than it would have been without compensation, they will continue to live with diseases, disabilities, and any loss of opportunities that lead caused. However, the decisions likely sent a deterrence message about consequences to companies causing lead exposure.

The significance of these tort cases is that although in many ways our public health laws and institutions failed these children and their families, another part of the legal system—the tort law—did redress some of their injuries. This is, however, a distant second best (or worse) to preventing the diseases and disabilities in the first place. During lectures on the tort law I often survey students or other audiences: Would they rather have some substantial compensation as the result of a tort case for the injuries they would have incurred and with which they would continue to live, or would they rather have never suffered the adverse effects at all? Unanimously, they opt for preventing the injuries instead of receiving postinjury compensation. Moreover, none of them likely have any idea of the process of bringing a tort suit, with all the anxiety, turmoil, and attention that might be involved.

To understand more about the tort law, we should ask some key questions. How well does it serve compensatory and deterrence functions? Since the tort law will have to address precisely the same kinds of chemical creations with which public health institutions struggle, how well does the tort law incorporate and utilize needed studies to successfully carry out its purposes?

INSTITUTIONAL TENDENCIES THAT AFFECT THE TORT LAW

In order for a citizen to receive redress for harm, she must have reasonable access to the law, and the procedures must give her a fair chance through legal procedures or processes to show the need for repairing the damage. That is, how the tort law functions, the kinds of wrongful actions that result in injuries, and the incentives of attorneys and experts to take legal cases should not be substantial hurdles for an attorney to file a case for action against alleged defendants. How does the tort law look on these dimensions?

To understand this issue, we distinguish between traumatic torts (sometimes called "private risk" torts) and "public risk" torts.

Clayton Gillette and James Krier provided a useful analysis of how the tort law might function in this area.

Private risks: " 'Private risks' . . . are either of natural origin or, if manmade, produced in relatively discrete units, with local impacts more or less subject to personal control." Traumatic risks, such as car accidents, are the examples I use.

In contrast, public-risk torts are "threats to human health or safety that are centrally or mass-produced, broadly distributed, and largely outside the individual risk bearer's direct understanding and control." These include things such as risks from toxic substances, nuclear accidents, pharmaceuticals, and contaminated products.[288]

Gillette and Krier discussed how access to the law and legal processes could affect legal outcomes. *Access* biases or tendencies (which I prefer) are "factors that work systematically for or against the interests of plaintiffs *as they seek to get their public risk claims into court in the first place*" (emphasis added).[289] *Process* biases or tendencies, in contrast, are institutional, "factors that work systematically for or against the interests of plaintiffs *once their public risk claims reach the courtroom*" (emphasis added).[290] These would include such things as the overall burden of proof, burdens of proof on particular issues, or other legal doctrines that make presenting a case easier or harder in court. Access tendencies might work for or against plaintiffs in bringing a case to court, while process tendencies can also work for or against plaintiffs once they are in court.

What are some access costs that injured parties face to bring cases for traumatic risk torts? Consider lawsuits to redress traumatic torts, such as automobile accidents. Even seeking compensation for these harms can be costly and risky because it takes the "investment of time and money, and success is hardly assured."[291] It is only when a plaintiff's expected legal judgments exceed, and perhaps substantially exceed, litigation costs that injured parties will likely seek access to the adjudication process.

Importantly, access costs for private, traumatic harms tend to be relatively low.[292] Car accident injuries are discrete; they appear at a particular time and place. Most injuries are obvious upon the accident. And a good many harms are readily recognizable (but not all, of course). Each of these features is accessible via our ordinary senses, reducing obstacles to recovery.

In addition, our understanding of accidents between large objects tends to ease the identification of defendants, the establishment of their liability, the demonstration of causation, and the proof of the dimensions of a plaintiff's loss. In general we know that one car colliding with another will cause damage to one or both. An accident sets in motion forces that can cause modest or substantial injuries to occupants in the cars or, less commonly, to bystanders. The effects of the forces that are generated are easily recognized and well understood.

Public risks: Access to the tort law to redress public risk harms is another matter. For example, harms may befall one from employment as a result of exposure to MOCA (4,4'-methylenebis [2-chloroaniline]). This substance is used in the polyurethane industry to create "tough, resistant polyurethane products."[293] These products become the basic material for "castable urethane rubber products such as shock-absorption pads and conveyor belting."[294] Laboratory scientists use it as a model for carcinogenicity, since it is a known human carcinogen.[295] People could similarly be harmed by drinking water contaminated by trichloroethylene (TCE), which is also a human carcinogen and a cause of Parkinson's disease, or by using it as a solvent in the workplace. What access hurdles might one face?

There are greater difficulties addressing harms from molecular invaders than those from largish physical objects typical of traumatic risks. Understanding and determining the risks from molecular substances are roughly analogous to the difficulties public health institutions have in diagnosing risks or harms from molecular invaders. (However, in principle, citizens may face greater hurdles in showing causation in the tort law to redress wrongs than public health agencies confront in establishing causation for preventive purposes.[296])

Diseases and dysfunctions triggered by molecular substances tend to be subtle, complicated, and often difficult to trace. On rare occasions, contact with a substance may cause a "signature disease," which is one that is "associated uniquely with exposure to an agent (e.g., asbestosis and exposure to asbestos),"[297] or one "that [is] uniquely related to exposure to a certain substance and [is] rarely observed in individuals that are not exposed."[298] Signature diseases tend to ease proof of harm and its source, but such obvious causal connections are quite rare.

Adverse health conditions might have several possible causal explanations. Scientists must identify which of several possible causes of disease is most likely. Multiple potential sources may complicate or confound the task of determining the real culprit.

Induction and latency periods of a disease may mask causal connections. In chapter 2, I noted a number of diseases that can be delayed months, years, or decades after toxic contacts occur, especially cancers. Identifying a person's disease because of childhood exposures would likely be particularly difficult.

When molecules contribute to harm, determining the extent of injury attributable to a particular exposure may be difficult. These problems are exacerbated if there are multiple possible contributors to the adverse effect. Which one caused how much of the harm?

Identifying a responsible defendant might be even more difficult, especially if toxic contributions come from the environment and no obvious agent disposed of the material. For example, there might be TCE in drinking water, but if the source is an underground aquifer, where did this solvent originate, how did it enter the groundwater, and who disposed of it?

Legal statutes of limitation might bar the initiation of a legal case. These are legal rules specifying that an injured party must file a legal case within a determinate period of time in order for it to be considered by the legal system. At one time, plaintiffs were required to file suits within a few years of *exposure* to a product that might have caused harm. However, long latency periods for some diseases could easily foreclose recovery because exposure might have occurred well before the disease appeared. Subsequently, most courts recognized a "discovery rule," which established that the legal clock does not start ticking until a plaintiff has discovered an injury.[299]

High costs and personal burdens of bringing a suit may reduce victims' incentives to sue and attorneys' incentives to take a case.[300] However, on this issue the costs of bringing a legal case may be different than the language suggests. Typically in tort suits a plaintiff need not pay the lawyer a retainer fee to take a case (and out of which fee the attorney would draw funds for work on the legal issues) or pay on an hourly basis. In most instances a person burdened by disease need not spend his or her own money trying to legally recoup losses caused by another.

Instead, in the United States, lawyers are typically compensated on a "contingent fee" basis. If plaintiff lawyers take a case, they agree to present it without charging the person who has been harmed up front. If the litigation is successful, the lawyer will take some percentage of the final settlement for his or her efforts, plus incurred expenses. However, if the case is not successful, the lawyer receives nothing—he or she must pay for experts' expenses and his or her own time out of the law firm's own or borrowed resources and receives nothing for the effort. Thus, cost issues would not typically be a problem for the person alleging injury. However, plaintiffs' lawyers can face important and risky business decisions: What are the chances of winning the case? Can I bring the case, pay all expenses, have a decent settlement for plaintiffs, and have money left over to pay for my time? Jonathan Haar's *A Civil Action* illustrates some of these issues.[301]

Consequently, lawyers have business reasons to screen injured parties and the cases they take. If legal costs would be substantial and their chances of winning are uncertain, lawyers might not take them. That said, some lawyers take toxic tort cases that seem dicey as business decisions because they believe in providing injured parties a chance to redress their injuries, even though succeeding in court might be difficult. One lawyer recently indicated that he earned about $0.75 per hour working on a case that resulted in a modest settlement for plaintiffs, a far cry from more-typical hourly fees of $300–$500 or more.

Plaintiffs themselves can have personal costs: time spent in participating on the case, time spent with lawyers providing information about exposure and other issues, and the personal anxiety of testifying under oath to opposing attorneys in depositions and in court. Some can even find a "stigma associated with the act of asserting a complaint, keeping the memory of the injury or loss alive, or continued confrontation with the injurer, a distressing prospect for most victims."[302] Together these concerns may be enough to discourage filing a suit.

Experts, too, can pose barriers to bringing a case. If the causal complexity is too great, the topic is outside one's expertise, or the right kind of legally required scientific evidence is not available, experts may not participate in a case. Sometimes lawyers might ask for testimony that an expert believes he or she cannot or should not provide. I know toxicological and medical experts who reject high percentages of cases in which they are asked to participate.

As a result, tort law access was much more difficult for "public" harms (e.g., exposures to toxicants) than for private/traumatic harms in 1990, when Gillette and Krier wrote their paper. Consequently, plaintiffs who believed they had been injured by chemical creations faced hurdles even in having their cases considered by the legal system. "When [such] claims go unfiled, the social costs they represent are not brought to bear on producer decision making. Because the signal emanating from the courts is thus weakened, there is likely to be too much public risk."[303] Thus, access barriers can diminish any deterrence the tort law might otherwise provide: as a result, "public risk litigation is probably marked by too few claims and too little vigorous prosecution, with the likely consequence that too much public risk escapes the deterrent effects of liability."[304]

Compensating process tendencies? Nonetheless, Gillette and Krier argued that access tendencies in public-risk cases were balanced by legal process or procedural tendencies that made success in a suit easier for plaintiffs once they were in court. They uneasily conceded a point of argument to others who had contended that "how claims are treated once they reach the courtroom" tends to favor plaintiffs.[305] The claim was that a few rules of liability tended to disfavor companies whose products posed risks to the public or workforce.

By accepting this tendentious point, Gillette and Krier ultimately—but cautiously—concluded that on balance the tort litigation system achieved optimum amount of risk even for public harms.[306] This concession was likely too optimistic in 1990 because it was far from clear that legal processes favored plaintiffs even at the time they wrote, since plaintiffs continued to have the burden of proof on all major issues. However, there had been a tiny number of cases, notably some concerning diethylstilbestrol (DES), that eased an occasional aspect of plaintiffs' proof burdens that critics overemphasized. These few cases were hardly representative of the entire tort law or toxic tort cases. Moreover, they were correct resolutions of the particular issues at stake.

HOW WELL DID THE TORT LAW FUNCTION IN 1992?

The year 1992 is a critical point in time for assessing the tort law. It was two years after Gillette and Krier published their analysis, Michael J. Saks had just compiled major social-science studies of torts, and it was one year before the *Daubert* decision modified scientific requirements in the law affecting both access and process tendencies. Saks's research revealed several major conclusions, some of which importantly bear on access and process tendencies of the tort law.[307]

Despite a common public narrative about the tort law—that too many people sue—in fact, few wrongfully injured people approach a lawyer or file a case for redress of harm. Evidence from medical malpractice cases illustrates these points.

A 1972 US Department of Health, Education, and Welfare study found that only about 6% of patients injured during medical care sought some kind of compensation for injuries, and only about 3% of these filed suits. A 1977 California Hospital Association study found that 10% of injured patients sought compensation but only one in six of those with "major, permanent" injuries filed suits (1.6% of all injured parties).[308]

A 1991 Rand study found that of every 100 people injured, 81% took no action at all. "Of the nineteen who considered making some sort of claim for compensation, two dealt directly with the injurer, four with the insurer, and seven consulted a lawyer (of whom four engaged the lawyer but only two filed suit); six did nothing. Thus, 87% are not heard from by the injurer or insurer, and only 2% become filed lawsuits."[309]

The Ohio Board of Medical Licensure and Discipline "found that only 1% of [parties with complaints about doctors] proceeded to file lawsuits."[310] Why is this? Some patients do not attribute responsibility for injuries, as would the law. Some patients do not know how to find a lawyer and initiate a case. Sometimes, injured parties "conduct an intuitive cost-benefit analysis of filing a lawsuit, including not only the dollar costs involved but the costs in time and stress associated with a suit" (this resembles points noted above).[311] Part of the explanation lies in the institution. "A system that requires victims to initiate claims and puts them through a complex process before compensation can be paid will have far fewer claims filed than a system that reduces these barriers."[312]

Consequently, Saks concludes that defendants are protected from facing legal liability because "victims tend not to complain."[313] Thus, the tort law's greatest error is that "an enormous number of persons who have been negligently injured will not receive the compensation that would be due them if they exercised their right to claim and had been able to find a lawyer willing to represent them. *Before the complaints are filed at the courthouse, defendants are billions of dollars ahead of where, under the law, they might expect to be*" (emphasis added).[314]

This research reinforces Gillette and Krier's point that tort law access has barriers. Some of this results from limitations in the evidence. Intimidation created by the institution, resulting in self-imposed reluctance by injured parties not to approach the law, or by nervousness created by participation in litigation further limit access. Although we sometimes hear about the fraudulent lawsuits, and there are some, the end result is that many wrongfully injured citizens never approach the tort law.

A further conclusion is that tort law also often poorly compensates people for their injuries. "From a compensation viewpoint, the problem with the tort system is not that it over-compensates or wildly compensates or imposes undue costs on liable injurers. Its principal shortcoming seems to be that it usually provides no compensation at all or, when it does, it under-compensates. So little compensation is achieved through the tort system that only as an act of hyperbole can it be said to be part of an injury compensation system."[315]

In 1992 the tort law surely functioned much less well in preventing and compensating injuries caused by public risks (e.g., industrial chemicals) than for traumatic torts, for the reasons Gillette and Krier provide. Despite their overall argument that access and process bias were optimally balanced, defendants in their activities and products probably underprotected the public.

THE 1993–1999 SEA CHANGE IN THE ADMISSIBILITY OF EXPERTS

Any balance between access and process tendencies for public risks that might have existed was upset beginning in 1993. In cases needing substantial scientific evidence, as litigation concerning public risks does, federal (and much state law) underwent a sea change following three Supreme Court decisions, noted earlier, that affect both access and process tendencies: *Daubert v. Merrell-Dow Pharmaceutical, Inc.* (1993), *General Electric v. Joiner* (1997), and *Kumho Tire v. Carmichael* (1999).

Until that time, courts had reviewed scientific testimony needed in tort cases under the so-called *Frye* rule issued by the U. S. Court of Appeals for the District of Columbia in 1923. As long as an expert was qualified to address the science at issue and was testifying about what a scientific test or procedure had shown, and the kind of test or procedure had been "generally accepted" by the relevant scientific community in which it was utilized, the expert could offer a professional *opinion* about what the science showed. This rule applied only to testimony relying on "new" or "novel" kinds of scientific studies; that is, new to a science field. Consequently, judges had a limited role in reviewing experts, and litigants had comparatively low barriers to introduce expert testimony into court.[316]

Under *Frye*, judges conducted only a generic review of novel studies about which an expert would testify—had the scientific community "generally accepted" the kind of study in question as scientifically reliable? Importantly, there was no inquiry into the particular *individual* testimony an expert would offer. In addition, if a jurisdiction had accepted "the [kind of] principle, technique, or test" about which an expert would testify, it became "established as a matter of law" and in the future would not be relitigated.[317] Opposing qualified experts could offer different opinions about the same studies. The *Frye* procedures fit well with an adversarial legal system—each side might have a different understanding of what the science showed, and *Frye* permitted both of them to testify to the jury. It would then decide which side's view of the science was more nearly correct.

Daubert v. Merrell Dow Pharmaceutical, Inc. (1993)[318]

In 1956 the Food and Drug Administration (FDA) authorized Merrell Dow to market a new pharmaceutical, Bendectin, designed to reduce morning sickness in pregnant women. However, sometime after Merrell Dow received approval to sell Bendectin, researchers and the FDA discovered that the company had hidden animal data that showed Bendectin caused birth defects quite similar to those of thalidomide (see chapter 1). Consequently, scientists and others developed some skepticism about the safety of Bendectin.[319] In turn, this unleashed a wave of concerns that led to additional research on Bendectin's connection to birth defects and then to a series of tort actions against Merrell Dow. Families in which pregnant women had taken Bendectin and whose children had been born with shortened limb defects brought suits for the injuries caused.

The *Daubert* plaintiffs, seeking compensation for the injuries of Jason Daubert and another child, Eric Schuller, presented the results of various kinds of scientific research regarding Bendectin's harmful effects on developing fetuses. This included "1) chemical structure activity analysis studies, 2) *in vitro* (test tube) studies, 3) *in vivo* (animal teratology) studies and 4) reanalysis of epidemiology studies" to show Bendectin caused shortened limbs.[320]

Plaintiffs' evidence should have satisfied previous interpretations of the *Frye* rule, permitting their experts to testify, because these *kinds of studies* were routinely used in science. However, defendants opposed plaintiffs' evidence with a number of human epidemiological studies that to varying degrees showed no statistically significant difference in shortened limb defects between children born to mothers who had taken Bendectin and those born to mothers who had not. Their argument? Evidence provided by human data was superior to that provided by the plaintiff's studies because it showed actual human impacts, and therefore the plaintiff's evidence should be excluded. The trial court agreed: a plethora of human epidemiological evidence trumped plaintiffs' substantial nonepidemiological evidence; the case was dismissed because there was insufficient evidence for the plaintiffs to go to a full jury trial.[321]

The Dauberts ultimately appealed this decision all the way to the US Supreme Court, losing at the U. S. Court of Appeals for the Ninth Circuit along the way.[322] The Supreme Court reversed the district and appellate court decisions, holding that the trial court had mistakenly used the *Frye* test for determining the admissibility of experts to testify to a jury. Thus, in a brief victory for plaintiffs, it also overturned the trial court's exclusion of plaintiffs' experts. The 1976 congressionally enacted Federal Rules of Evidence (FRE) superseded *Frye*. On remand to the lower courts, the Ninth Circuit ruled that even under the new rules, plaintiffs did not have sufficient evidence for their experts to testify to a jury.[323]

Unfortunately, the Supreme Court's Janus-faced opinion occasioned some difficulties. One face liberalized the admission of expert testimony, which tended to favor plaintiffs and to assist protecting the public's health through the tort law—namely, that the "[*Frye* rule's] austere [and rigid] standard ... would be at odds with the 'liberal thrust' of the revised FRE and their 'general approach of relaxing the traditional barriers to 'opinion' testimony.'"[324] An expert's testimony need have only "a reliable [scientific] foundation and [be] relevant to the task at hand."[325] While this reasoning required a better scientific foundation for expert testimony and a greater judicial role than under *Frye*, it might not have unduly burdened litigants' expert witnesses in presenting testimony.

Daubert simultaneously presented a different mien. The Supreme Court sought to describe how judges should review expert testimony and scientific evidence that could be presented to a jury. Despite the FRE's "liberalizing" features, a judge had a "gatekeeping" role in reviewing expert testimony. Judges now had increased duties to review scientific studies and to determine if an expert's testimony was both "reliable" and "relevant" to the issues of the case. Judges' roles were substantially enhanced and more intrusive in the legal process than they had been under the *Frye* rule.

What problems did this pose? Justice Harry Blackmun, writing for the Court, perhaps unintentionally used language that created new openings for defendants to argue that the plaintiffs' expert witnesses should not be allowed to testify in toxic tort trials. In an effort to explain that all expert testimony must rest on research properly grounded in science, Blackmun ventured to elucidate reliable science. Drawing on various amicus briefs, he wrote about scientific testimony that was founded on scientific "theories," "principles," "techniques," and "methodology," and that had "error rates" that could be determined and that had been peer reviewed, "tested," and published. His general, fairly abstract linguistic expressions seemed to apply as much to expert *testimony* as to the underlying *studies* that support testimony, but these are quite different.

His language in effect invited defendants to challenge not only the scientific research that plaintiffs proposed as evidence, but also the reliability of the testimony itself on various grounds. Defense lawyers began to ask whether plaintiffs' experts' *testimony* (in contrast to the studies by which the testimony was supported) had been tested, peer reviewed, or published or had an acceptable error rate. If testimony did not meet these particular standards, it should not be presented.

This can and likely did mislead judges, moving some of them to dismiss cases because testimony did not satisfy requirements more appropriate for *studies*. Improperly used, the *Daubert* requirements can mistakenly exclude quite proper scientific testimony. On a few occasions when I have testified in court, defense lawyers have asked me precisely some of these questions about scientists' testimony in the case.

The Court might not have foreseen how trial lawyers would use its decision. Indeed, at the end of its opinion, it returned to the idea of more-liberal rules for admitting expert testimony for juries' consideration: a trial court should admit some expert testimony that might be weakly supported by scientific studies. Rather than preventing juries from hearing the testimony, "shaky but admissible evidence" should be subjected to the "traditional and appropriate means" by which the validity of evidence and testimony are challenged in courts of law; namely, "(v)igorous cross-examination, presentation of contrary evidence, and careful instruction on the burden of proof."[326]

Justice Blackmun's excursion into the philosophy of science gave defense lawyers grounds for misleading challenges to the science, which some trial judges accepted and which made it more difficult for plaintiffs to present expert testimony based on new forms of toxicological research.

Finally, an unfortunate remnant from the *Daubert* cases nationwide likely left courts and defense attorneys with the idea that statistically based human epidemiological studies were the best or, as some courts said, the *only* kind of evidence that could show a substance could cause adverse human harm.[327] In the Bendectin litigation, a large number of human epidemiological studies showed no effect between a mother's use of Bendectin and her child being born with shortened limbs.

Consequently, what the courts saw as excellent evidence in this case ultimately created bad law in other courts. The reason? Epidemiological studies, readily available and easy to conduct in the Bendectin cases, are less easy to conduct for other exposures and may not even be available in many cases in which citizens have been wrongly injured. (Moreover, it is not clear whether the trial court recognized that "no evidence of adverse effects" does not imply "evidence of no adverse effects.") This residue of having good epidemiological evidence posed problems for a considerable period of time (see chapter 4).

Because of *Daubert* (1993), *judges* are now the arbiters of admissible individual scientific testimony, assessing whether or not the "general acceptance" of a *kind* of study is insufficient. They must determine if an expert's scientific testimony is derived by a "reliable" methodology—supported by appropriate scientific data—and is "relevant" to the facts of the case.[328]

The reaction to the original *Daubert* decision was mixed. Many commentators, the defense bar, and even some plaintiffs' lawyers and experts hailed it. *Daubert* had ushered in an era in which the law would better conform to relevant scientific research related to legal cases. This general response was soon tempered as critical scholarly articles following *Daubert* and *Joiner* began to appear, discussing their shortcomings and how they were being applied.[329]

Unfortunately, the legal ramifications of an epidemiological requirement led lower courts to insist on such studies, something that distinguished scientific committees would not necessarily require for identifying human health hazards. Of course, human health studies can offer good evidence of adverse effects in humans, if they are well conducted (more on this in chapter 4), but often they cannot be. Epidemiology is an "inherently conservative" approach to causation that defendants were urging upon judges, and many of them accepted it.[330] In addition, critics argued that trial and appellate judges had subtly modified existing law on causation by increasing the threshold of scientific proof, and by making legal rules about types and strengths of scientific evidence."[331]

General Electric v. Joiner (1997)[332]

Four years later in *General Electric v. Joiner*, the Supreme Court took an appeal, largely on a procedural point about the appropriate standard an appellate court should follow in reviewing a trial court's decision to admit or exclude expert testimony.[333] Its decision erected another evidentiary barrier for plaintiffs in tort suits involving toxic chemicals.

At the district court level, Mr. Joiner, a 37-year-old erstwhile smoker with a family history of lung cancer, claimed that his exposure to polychlorinated biphenyls (PCBs) and some derivatives—dioxins and furans—promoted his lung cancer, from which he ultimately died before litigation was finalized. The trial judge, following defendants' arguments, individually examined four of thirteen epidemiological studies and two animal studies on which Joiner's expert testimony was based. She found each study to be *individually* insufficient to support the plaintiffs' ultimate scientific conclusion.

Mr. Joiner appealed the judge's evidentiary ruling to the U.S. Court of Appeals for the Eleventh Circuit, arguing that the judge should have considered the body of evidence as a whole from which scientists could infer the best explanation for what occurred. The Eleventh Circuit agreed with the plaintiffs' reasoning and reinstated the case for trial. However, the Eleventh Circuit also reasoned that it would more closely review trial decisions that precluded expert testimony that ended a legal case. Following this decision, defendants appealed to the Supreme Court, which overturned the Eleventh Circuit on this procedural point.

Of greater concern, the Supreme Court upheld the trial judge's study-by-study evaluation of each piece or line of evidence for whether it supported the plaintiff's ultimate causal conclusion. The district court could properly "conclude that the studies upon which [the plaintiff's] experts relied were not sufficient, whether individually or in combination, to support their conclusions . . . [that it] did not abuse its discretion in excluding their testimony."[334]

While the Supreme Court reviewed the trial court's analysis of individual studies on which plaintiffs relied, it did not analyze whether the total body of evidence supported the claim that PCB exposure contributed to Joiner's lung cancer. Justice John Paul Stevens dissented from this part of Court's argument.

The Court's failure to recognize and assess Joiner's total body of evidence has invited considerable critique. An important one came from the Federal Judicial Center's *Reference Manual on Scientific Evidence*, which provides a guide to courts in their review of scientific evidence and expert testimony. The law essay argued that the "slicing-and-dicing approach" endorsed by the *Joiner* Court to assess the validity of scientific evidence and testimony was contrary to how well-respected and prestigious scientific bodies, such as the International Agency for Research on Cancer (IARC), the National Research Council (NRC), and the National Institute for Environmental Health Sciences, determine which hypothesis is best supported by a body of evidence.[335] The *Joiner* decision subsequently led defense lawyers to try to undermine the plaintiffs' expert testimony by adopting a narrow conception of scientific evidence and the largely unscientific reasoning for evaluating it.

Scientists in fact consider a total body of relevant scientific evidence to determine adverse health effects on people. Moreover, they should be permitted to do so in court.[336] Shortly after the *Joiner* decision, philosopher of science Susan Haack pointed out how central plaintiffs' argument strategy is in science. She highlighted the reasoning in one of the most important scientific papers in biology in 60 years, perhaps the most important one in the 20th century—James Watson and Francis Crick's justly famous paper on the double-helix structure of DNA.[337]

> Sometimes bits of evidence which are individually weak are jointly strong; sometimes not—it depends what they are, and whether or not they reinforce each other (whether or not the crossword entries interlock). Chargaff's discovery that there are approximate regularities in the relative proportions of adenine and thymine, guanine and cytosine in DNA is hardly, by itself, strong evidence that DNA is a double-helical, backbone-out macromolecule with like-with-unlike base pairs; Franklin's X-ray photographs of the B form of DNA are hardly, by themselves, strong evidence that DNA is a double-helical, backbone-out macromolecule with like-with-unlike base pairs. That the tetra-nucleotide hypothesis is false is hardly, by itself, strong evidence that DNA is a double-helical, backbone-out macromolecule with like-with-unlike base pairs; and so on. But put all these pieces of evidence together, and the double-helical, backbone-out, like-with-unlike base pairs, structure of DNA is very well-warranted indeed (in fact, the only entry that fits).[338]

Because of the centrality of such arguments to scientists' reasoning, I note various uses of them in chapter 4. In fact the *Joiner* Court appears to err in its assessment.[339]

Kumho Tire v. Carmichael (1999)[340]

In a third case on admitting expert testimony, the Supreme Court held that the FRE apply to all expert testimony, including that of "practical" experts, which involved a tire inspection expert in this case. More importantly, the court's ruling provides important guidance to lower courts in how they should review expert testimony. The court, reinforcing greater convergence between legal decisions and pertinent scientific evidence from the scientific field, held that its gatekeeping requirement "is to make certain that an expert . . . employs in the courtroom the same level of intellectual rigor that characterizes the practice of an expert in the relevant field."[341]

The Court then further explained this point; the plaintiffs' expert's testimony about tire defects was excluded because it "fell outside the range where experts might reasonably differ, and where the jury must decide among the conflicting views of different experts, even though the evidence is 'shaky.'"[342] This most important heuristic can guide courts in reviewing expert testimony, which clarifies *Daubert* and to a large extent ameliorates some problems occasioned by *Joiner*. I return to it in chapter 4.

HOW WELL DID THE TORT LAW PROTECT CITIZENS FROM PUBLIC RISKS IN 2010?

After the effects of the *Daubert, Joiner,* and *Kumho Tire* cases pervaded the legal system, how had they changed the litigation of public risks since 1990, when Gillette and Krier wrote? *Daubert* and *Joiner* as applied (sometimes mistakenly) by lower courts increased both access and procedural barriers for plaintiffs, reducing chances of their experts to address the jury and reducing the deterrence that comes from successful tort suits.

First, litigants' expert witnesses, and especially plaintiffs', must pass an increasingly stringent review to have experts testify (procedural), which decreases access (because of costs, lawyer screening, and expert screening). There are several facets to this. Judges have a duty to review individual expert testimony, and often there is a mini "Daubert" hearing before the judge at which litigants present and challenge each other's experts. Plaintiffs typically face the greatest scrutiny because they have the burden of proof to present enough evidence for a court to justify impaneling a jury to decide the issues.

Access is also affected because lawyers must ensure that they have good witnesses (as they always needed) and that witnesses are properly prepared both for depositions and a hearing before a judge. All this takes more time and money than previously, increasing pre-trial costs. Thus, lawyers must be more cautious in accepting cases.

Second, there are now more procedural hurdles for lawyers and experts to go through before an actual legal case can be presented to a jury. Moreover, judges' reviews of scientific testimony created a procedural hurdle that did not exist under *Frye*. This increases both legal effort and costs for lawyers and experts.

Third, in implementing *Daubert* and *Joiner* a number of courts have erred in reviewing expert testimony, asymmetrically affecting plaintiffs because they have the main burden of proof. Some judges have insisted that testimony must be based on certain kinds of evidence that might be ideal, as *Daubert* courts urged (e.g., epidemiological studies), but are not necessary to draw conclusions about toxic effects of substances on people. Other courts placed special legal requirements on epidemiological studies, increasing procedural barriers.

Some courts mistakenly prevented experts' reliance on evidence that scientists would normally use, such as animal studies, human case studies, chemical structure–biological activity relationships, and mechanistic data, as scientifically insufficient to support an expert's conclusion. This especially occurred when there were no human epidemiological studies. Yet, an appropriate combination of such data can be quite sufficient for certain toxicity judgments. I consider these issues further in chapter 4.[343]

If plaintiffs' experts do not have a legally recognized scientific foundation for testimony, they may not testify to a jury. Invariably this means that a plaintiff's case is at an end.

Courts have also had difficulty understanding the nature of scientific reasoning—what philosophers would call an inference to the best explanation, or a weight-of-the-evidence argument. I return to this point at the end of this chapter and in chapter 4.[344] Mistaken trial court decisions on admitting scientific experts are more difficult to appeal and even more difficult to overturn because of the *Joiner* and *Kumho Tire* cases.

As a result, courts have tended to asymmetrically exclude plaintiffs' experts because they judged the scientific support was insufficient. Although the *Daubert* line of decisions applies to all legal cases needing expert testimony, including those in the criminal law, it has been most stringently enforced in the tort law. In criminal cases, district or appellate courts have not for the most part precluded scientific evidence and testimony, often based on notoriously unreliable evidence (despite what TV shows suggest) poorly grounded in scientific studies.

In 2000 the *New York Times* reported a study reviewing the effects of *Daubert* and its progeny on the tort law. "[T]he number of product-liability cases filed in federal court has dropped by more than half the last four years, from 32,856 in 1997 [the year of the *Joiner* decision] to 14,428 in 2000 . . . a reflection, some legal scholars say, of how selective many lawyers have become."[345] This forced many plaintiffs' lawyers to buttress "their arguments with platoons of experts, and improv[e] their chances of winning by choosing only truly egregious cases involving the most seriously injured parties."[346] "If they're not a quadriplegic, a paraplegic or losing some part of their body, there's no way I'm going to take that case," as one lawyer, Craig Hilborn, put it.[347] Tort cases had become "increasingly expensive to bring, often costing well above $100,000."[348]

Anecdotal evidence now suggests that this woefully underestimates plaintiffs' costs, especially in complex cases, where they can be as high as $1 million.[349] In addition, as much as 60% of the cost of a plaintiff's case might occur before trial begins. If plaintiffs' experts are not admitted, then there will be no trial and these costs would be wasted. This raises the stakes on a lawyer's business decision, for which Hilborn's comments are perhaps representative.

A 2013 review of four million cases found that "the adoption of *Daubert* in federal court did, in a statistically significant manner, motivate defendants to remove their cases from more plaintiff friendly states using the *Frye* rules to federal jurisdictions using *Daubert* and its progeny that tend to be more friendly to defendants."[350] It also redirected where plaintiffs seek to bring cases.[351] These studies substantiate previous assessments in law review articles. Because defendants find the sea change on scientific testimony much more attractive, they go to jurisdictions where their chances of success are enhanced.

While the federal implementation of *Daubert* and associated cases has precluded numerous plaintiffs seeking redress for exposures to toxic substances from trial, because courts have in effect made scientific mistakes, I close this chapter by pointing to a major case decided by the U. S. Court of Appeals for the First Circuit that holds the promise of correcting some prominent misunderstandings of the law and science needed in toxic tort cases.

HOPE FOR BETTER PROTECTIONS: *MILWARD V. ACUITY SPECIALTY PRODUCTS*[352]

We met Brian Milward in the introduction; he alleged that benzene had caused his quite rare acute promyelocytic leukemia (APL).

However, because there were no good human epidemiological studies that his expert, toxicologist Martyn Smith of the University of California, Berkeley, could use in support of his testimony, he had to rely on various lines of data to show that benzene could cause APL in humans.

As a result, the Milwards' lawyer, Steve Jensen, contacted me to articulate and substantiate the methodology that Smith was using—an inference to the best explanation, or what scientists often call a weight-of-the-evidence argument (see the reference to Haack's landmark article earlier in this chapter). I had long argued in research that courts should allow experts to use this form of argument because it is so commonly used by scientists in various fields.[353] Professor Smith had used such an inference to conclude that benzene could cause APL.[354] Martyn's and my tasks in the *Milward* case were to persuade the trial judge to admit Martyn to present his testimony to a jury, to make the assertion that exposure to benzene more likely than not could cause APL. We both failed.

As noted in the introduction, district court judge O'Toole excluded Martyn's testimony, and the Milwards' attempt at redress for Mr. Milward's APL was at an end in district court. The Milwards appealed their trial court loss to the US Court of Appeals for the First Circuit.

I claimed in the introduction that there was overwhelming evidence that the Milwards were treated unjustly. Why did I make such a strong claim? How Judge O'Toole reviewed the Milwards' scientific evidence and his choices in assessing it were mistaken and have implications for whether or not Mr. Milward received proper redress for his disease. My assertion has good support from the appellate ruling on the evidence (and on my judgment about the correctness of the appellate court's assessment of the evidence and Smith's argument).

A major theme of this book is that how science is used in the law can determine whether or not the citizens under public heath laws or plaintiffs in tort cases are treated justly or not. This case illustrates an important aspect of the theme.

The First Circuit accepted the Milwards' appeal and overturned the trial court. Other federal circuits, district courts, and the West Virginia Supreme Court have adopted aspects of the First Circuit's decision.[355] Michael D. Green, a well-known legal scholar, calls this decision "one of the most significant toxic tort cases in recent memory." I believe that this court came to the correct conclusions both about the science and the law.

First, the First Circuit found that trial judge O'Toole had made a legal mistake—in legal argot, he *abused his authority* in his ruling. There is a strict line between the role of judge as gatekeeper of *reliable and relevant testimony* and the jury's role as finder of fact to determine the *correctness of scientific issues*, a line Judge O'Toole mistakenly crossed.[356] The court also held that the proponents of scientific testimony—either plaintiffs or defendants—need not prove to the trial judge that an expert's presentation of scientific evidence is *correct*, but only "that the expert's conclusion has been arrived at in a scientifically sound and methodologically reliable fashion.'"[357] In a number of earlier federal cases, trial judges appeared to be doing precisely this—trying to determine which side's evidence was correct instead of assessing whether or not the evidence and testimony met a sufficient standard to be presented to a jury.

Second, following the *Kumho Tire* case, the First Circuit additionally held that a trial judge is not permitted to take sides between experts whose views exhibit the same intellectual rigor in court as in their fields.[358] If reasonable scientists have different views of a possible cause of a disease, a trial judge may not "determine which of several competing scientific theories has the best provenance."[359]

Moreover, because Judge O'Toole seemed to join the scientific debate when he "repeatedly challenged the factual underpinnings of Dr. Smith's opinion, and took sides on questions . . . on which reasonable scientists can clearly disagree . . . the court overstepped the authorized bounds of its role as gatekeeper."[360] These errors, one might say, are attributable to the district court judge not fully grasping his limited legal role. The First Circuit explicitly clarified it.

Third, the appellate court also found that Judge O'Toole did not properly evaluate the scientific evidence and the weight-of-the-evidence argument presented by Smith and supported by my foundation. "At times, the court's error in excluding Dr. Smith's testimony derived from a mistake in its understanding of the weight of the evidence methodology. . . . The court treated the separate evidentiary components of Dr. Smith's analysis atomistically, as though his ultimate opinion was *independently* supported by each."[361] Smith's testimony was based on five different lines of evidence from the peer-reviewed literature.[362] "As explained by plaintiffs' expert on methodology Dr. Cranor, Distinguished Professor of Philosophy at the University of California, Riverside, inference to the best explanation can be thought of as involving six general steps, some of which may be implicit. The scientist must 1) identify an association between an exposure and a disease, 2) consider a range of plausible explanations for the association, 3) rank the rival explanations according to their plausibility, 4) seek additional evidence to separate the more plausible from the less plausible explanations, 5) consider all of the relevant available evidence, and 6) integrate the evidence using professional judgment to come to a conclusion about the best explanation."[363]

In strong language the First Circuit added, "No serious argument can be made that the weight of the evidence approach is inherently unreliable. Rather, admissibility must turn on the particular facts of the case . . ."[364] The important question was this: Did "Dr. Smith, in reaching his opinion, [apply] the methodology with "the same level of intellectual rigor" that he uses in his scientific practice?"[365] The First Circuit ruled he had.

The First Circuit correctly found that this form of argument is central to drawing conclusions from several different lines of scientific evidence. This holding is important for the law. For some time after a 1994 decision in the U.S. Court of Appeals for the Fifth Circuit ruled against plaintiffs' weight-of-the-evidence reasoning, other courts were tempted to follow it. A common defense strategy then was to argue that plaintiffs' experts should not be permitted to use this form of reasoning to present evidence. The First Circuit saw the significance of such arguments in science, thus providing a much-needed and valuable counter to the Fifth Circuit's claim. Had this court not endorsed the use of these arguments, it would have handicapped scientists to near testimonial impotence because inferences to the best explanation are standard in many fields (see chapter 4).

Nonetheless, defendants continue to denigrate and caricature them because of the role of professional judgment in them. Here is an extreme statement from a well-known defense attorney: "Take all the evidence, throw it into the hopper, close your eyes, open your heart, and guess the weight. You could be a lucky winner!"[366]

The First Circuit, as if anticipating such comments, strongly differs: the role of judgment in the weight-of-the-evidence approach "does not mean that the approach is any less scientific. . . . [Any] 'evaluation of data and scientific evidence to determine whether an inference of causation is appropriate requires judgment and interpretation.'"[367]

As a fourth point, the First Circuit also sharply disagreed with Judge O'Toole's view "that although epidemiological evidence is not always essential," the defendants were "correct that sound epidemiological studies are ordinarily needed to confirm, by consistent observation, an hypothesis of causation."[368] The First Circuit pointed out the flaw: "The district court read too much into the paucity of statistically significant epidemiological studies. The absence of peer-reviewed epidemiological studies does not, as defendants contend, make it 'almost impossible' for Dr. Smith's opinion to be admissible. Epidemiological studies are not per se required as a condition of admissibility regardless of context."[369] In this holding, the court endorsed well-entrenched views from distinguished scientific committees that assess adverse health effects from toxicants (see chapter 4).

THE AFTERMATH OF *MILWARD*

The defendants appealed the First Circuit decision to the US Supreme Court, but the Court rejected the appeal without comment, as is typical in cases where appeals are not accepted.[370] When the case was returned to the district court of origin, the First Federal District of Massachusetts assigned a new judge for the remaining issues in the case. Most of 22 defendants settled; a few could show that Mr. Milward had no benzene exposure from their products. One remaining defendant challenged the Milwards on one remaining issue that is currently in process.

Importantly, Brian Milward is alive. He has not succumbed to his benzene-caused APL as of this date. Also, he likely received substantial compensation from the companies that settled, but, as is typical, settlement details have not been disclosed. Even though his cancer is in remission, the aftereffects of the treatment and the cancer are not necessarily pleasant.

Nearly a decade of chemotherapy, along with diabetes and a rare bowel disorder, have left him battling what he calls "absolutely ridiculous" fatigue. Retired and on disability, he remembers returning to work twice. First, he resorted to napping to endure an eight-hour shift. When his boss assigned him to office duty, pushing paper and making calls, he still fell asleep at his desk.

"I can't really do anything," said Milward, 57—at least, not what he loves: repairing race cars, working in his yard, playing with his grandchildren. "It just sucks when you get a cancer like this."[371]

The outcome of Mr. Milward's case illustrates some important points about the legal system. First, public health laws failed him because companies were permitted to produce products containing sufficiently high levels of benzene that he contracted APL. Better screening of products for toxic ingredients and their permissible concentrations before they enter commerce might have better protected him, but, of course, this is difficult to determine.

Second, the tort law, backing up regulatory failures, worked well for him—finally. It took seven years from the time he contracted APL until he had a favorable decision on general causation, and four years from the time he and his wife filed suit against the defendant companies until he received favorable settlements.

He did receive some, perhaps substantial, redress for his disease. His settlements have probably helped with or fully paid for medical bills associated with his cancer and have provided some recompense for the hardship and misery he has been through. Has he been adequately compensated? I do not know. In general, according to Michael Saks the tort law at the low end of costs overcompensates people for injuries suffered but tends to undercompensate people for injuries in excess of $100,000 (in 1992 dollars).[372]

Even though the legal system provided redress for his injuries, thanks to a wise decision by the First Circuit Court of Appeals, Mr. Milward has not been made whole. His health has not returned to its condition before he contracted APL. Mr. Milward's disease substantially truncated his opportunity range compared to a healthy 57-year-old American male. The pertinent public health law and companies' behavior caused injuries to him. Because he has difficulty playing with grandchildren, myriad other activities will be unavailable. He cannot work at even the physically easiest jobs. He cannot play tennis. He cannot go hiking. He cannot celebrate his 60th birthday by climbing a 14,000- or 19,000-foot-high mountain. He likely cannot swim in a pool or the ocean. He may not even be able to stay awake for normal periods of time. Thus, *even with favorable tort law redress*, his opportunity range has shrunk substantially.

Imagine how he would assess the justice of his circumstances had he not received redress in torts. If Judge O'Toole's decision had controlled his fate, Mr. Milward would have been treated unjustly in myriad ways. Even before the tort case, he likely experienced legal battery because he was unknowingly exposed to the carcinogen benzene; there was no alert that it was in products he used. Public health laws did not prevent benzene in those products from causing his APL. Had he not received redress from the tort law, he would have been denied compensation for his medical expenses and injuries. This would have resulted in multiple injustices toward him, without compensation for these costs and perhaps without sufficient medical treatment and compensation. He might well have had increased misery associated with his disease. This would have been added to the Milwards' tragedy. Fortunately, the First Circuit understood the issues and decided them correctly, and Mr. Milward received redress for his injuries. Yet, he had been treated unjustly in several ways up to that point.

CONCLUSION

Obscure Supreme Court decisions and their implementation in lower courts have already affected numerous litigants and will continue to do so. Some courts construed scientific evidence and reasoning contrary to good scientific practice as exemplified by distinguished scientific committees. Courts so ruled despite the Supreme Court's aim that experts employ "in the courtroom the same level of intellectual rigor that characterizes the practice of an expert in the relevant field."[373] I develop these points further in chapter 4.

Such decisions are likely traceable to several things: complex patterns of evidence and the substantive relevance of some evidence, opponents' oversimplifications and obfuscations of the science, and the ambiguity of the *Daubert* decision. Courts also have struggled with scientific evidence and testimony, both of which are substantially outside their normal education. They may have overreacted to some language in *Daubert*, to *Joiner's* endorsement of an atomistic analysis of data, or to the "intellectual rigor" language in *Kumho Tire*, while not noticing the Court's gloss that expert opinions are admissible if they fall within "the range where experts might reasonably differ, and where the jury must decide among the conflicting views of different experts, even though the evidence is 'shaky.'"[374] Finally, the complexity of inferences to the best explanation may have caused problems.

In order to address scientific issues better in the future, judges will need to recognize the complexity of scientific reasoning, understand the wide range of evidentiary patterns that scientists themselves employ to infer causation, and provide for a wider range of reasonable scientific disagreements than some have done to date.[375] The *Milward* decision did all this consistent with the Supreme

Court's decisions in *Daubert, Joiner*, and *Kumho Tire*. If other courts follow the First Circuit's lead, this will allow scientists to testify in the courtroom as they would in their fields, reduce some process barriers for plaintiffs, perhaps increase some access for plaintiffs and lawyers, increase the possibility of justice for plaintiffs, and help make the world a somewhat safer place through modest deterrence advances.

Before the *Milward* decision, some plaintiffs, unlike Brian Milward, had lesser chances for redress for harms they had suffered. Companies whose products may have harmed them would be among hundreds or thousands who were millions of dollars ahead of where they should have been legally, because judicial decisions on scientific issues were mistakenly decided in their favor.[376] An improper deterrence message would have resulted from the legal outcome—those companies' conduct would not have been judged as legally wrong. Risky practices and products might have continued as they had before. Thus, there would have been no deterrence by example or by reform. Ordinary citizens likely would have continued at a heightened risk from other companies.

In contrast, subsequent to *Milward* some important deterrence-by-example and deterrence-by-reform messages have reinforced the tort law's general discouragement of risky activities. Companies that incorporate benzene (or perhaps other toxicants) in their products might well modify them, highlight warnings, or make existing warnings easier to understand. Indeed, benzene is quite dangerous. The *Milward* case showed that while one product's use might or might not have caused Mr. Milward's APL, the multiple products containing benzene to which he was exposed could and did cause his disease. Even so, acute promyelocytic leukemia substantially transformed his life—he says it "sucks." After contracting and treating APL, his range of lifetime opportunities has been substantially truncated.

Chapter 4

How Demands for Ideal Science Undermine the Public's Health

INTRODUCTION

Postmarket public health laws aim to "prevent" diseases and dysfunctions in children and adults, but these laws do so inadequately. The absence of premarket toxicity testing plus postexposure, postviolation responses to risks create and invite ignorance about substances and can cause harm, misery, and injustice. Consequently, legislative choices about *when* science is utilized are important legal and social decisions. Science used to determine the toxicity before products enter commerce is the best way to protect the public (see chapter 2 and below), as Congress has just endorsed.

However, the 1976 TSCA and other postmarket laws that governed current chemical products in commerce create incentives for a less visible and deeper problem with the science-law interaction: *how much* and *what kind of* scientific studies are required to reduce or remove risks to protect the public? Legal requirements and informal pressures to demand too many or repetitive scientific studies can result from certain ideal but unwise scientific views in the law. The more kinds of studies that are required to substantiate the toxicity of each product, the more this slows the analysis of the substance in question and precludes considering a large number of unevaluated products. This will continue ignorance about the toxicity of substances and exacerbate injustices. For contrast, this chapter also briefly suggests how science in such circumstances could be better used to protect the public. (The issues in this chapter are largely separable from the dishonorable uses of science discussed in chapter 1.)

A similar problem arises in the tort law, although there are some differences. For one thing, the tort law is necessarily a post-exposure, post harm part of the legal system, entering people's lives only after harm has occurred. However, it can have some favorable future deterrent effects. For another, judges screen experts before they can testify in front of juries, but judges typically do not decide final scientific issues. For a third thing, the tort law has much less uniform approaches to science than public health agencies. The reason: 678 federal district court judges administer first-level tort trials, and about 179 judges in federal courts of appeal review decisions of district courts. Nine Supreme Court justices who decide about 100 cases each year are the final appeal, if they take a case. Appellate courts provide some degree of uniformity (certainly within each circuit) by adjudicating lower-court decisions. Nonetheless, individual trial decisions about scientific data and testimony might still be more varied than the science used in public health actions because judges have considerable discretion within precedents.[377]

This chapter focuses on "how much" and "what kind" of science is required in the domains of postmarket public health law and tort law, respectively. Companies and pressures from politicians and lobbyists likely urge too much, even "ideal" science compared with what might be needed to prudently protect the public. Thus, ideal science (or science without any "doubt") can become the enemy of sufficient data to protect the public. (This can also be exacerbated by administrative procedures that public health agencies must follow.) Acceding to their demands will continue and exacerbate recklessness toward citizen's health and will treat them unjustly.[378]

Under public health laws, the best protections would come from premarket toxicity testing and review specifically tailored for the task, as some National Academy of Sciences committees have suggested (more below), I have argued, and Congress has now recognized. This also resembles REACH, a law adopted in the European Union (see chapter 2). Failing that, once products are in commerce, better use of science and monitoring of the public and workers' health could improve information generation, somewhat increase protections, and is reasonably possible. However, these efforts would have limitations in improving the public's health.

In the tort law, judges also must make important choices about how to administer the science needed in support of corrective justice. Both trial and appellate judges could make it more or less difficult for injured parties to present their cases to juries by *how much* and *what kinds of* scientific support they require. Demanding too much or misguided science may close off a party's chance at redress and undermine deterrence messages. Permitting too little might increase plaintiffs' chances for success but result in mistaken final messages if juries err. Courts should make judicious choices in guiding the science in court, but once testimony is presented to a jury, their ultimate decisions are more of a gamble. The *Milward* case from the First Circuit Court of Appeals provides a good guide to these issues, to which I return below.

Finally, both areas of the law can importantly issue *authoritative findings* about whether or not substances pose risks. Before a public health agency has made a toxicity finding and improved health protections for a substance, citizens may be unsure about how risky, for example, formaldehyde, C8, TCE, flame retardants, phthalates, or bisphenol A are. Should people try to avoid them as best they can or bury their heads and not worry about them? If there have been no authoritative findings, are exposures safe for people? We know that numerous substances are risky (chapter 2), yet there have been few legal actions to better protect the public's health—authoritative scientific statements have been in short supply.

The tort law has a similar role in issuing authoritative findings. If a trial court concludes that a defendant's exposure harmed the plaintiff(s), this sends a message that the product is a threat to one's health in similar circumstances. In contrast, if a tort jury finds that an exposure does not harm the plaintiffs, this communicates that the product is safer than some had worried, at least for that particular context.[379] Appellate court decisions affirming or overturning lower-court decisions are even more crucially authoritative.

HOW IDEAL SCIENCE IN PUBLIC HEALTH INSTITUTIONS CAN FOSTER IGNORANCE AND INJUSTICE

If public health institutions must provide the most complete and scientifically certain evidence of adverse effects to reduce risks, this will extend the public's ignorance even about toxic products and their own unjust treatment. To see this, consider a theoretical point, something of a scientific ideal.

Arthur Furst, a well-known and broadly educated toxicologist, argued for a rich and substantial scientific database in order to substantiate a chemical as a *human* carcinogen. *As a scientist* he sought to ensure that a substance was a human carcinogen. He was not making proposals either for regulatory agencies or for the tort law.

He urged the following:

> As an absolute minimum, there should be a close agreement
> between conclusions from well-designed epidemiological stud-
> ies of exposed populations, with conclusions drawn from good
> and valid animal bioassays (using appropriate routes of expo-
> sure and reasonable exposure levels and with an end point
> in which a cancer has been induced, one similar to that of the
> exposed human). Some corroboration from short-term tests will
> strengthen the association. If the biotransformation of the agent
> under consideration is similar in humans and on active animal
> species, there are more reasons to consider this agent a human
> carcinogen. The limitation is that the mechanism of action of the
> agent in inducing an animal cancer does not undergo a process
> or require an organ for which there is no human counterpart.[380]

This scientific ideal ensures that a chemical creation is a human
carcinogen. For protecting the public, one must be concerned about
what constitutes *sufficient* scientific data for the task, taking into
account the kinds of evidence available, the effects of higher and
lower exposures, and susceptible subpopulations such as children.
Considerations of justice suggest we should not adopt Professor
Furst's recommendations; they are unwise for postmarket laws and
for torts, but his views do provide a useful foil for our discussion.

In addressing a substance and whether or not it is toxic, we
could be ignorant, or "dumb" (to borrow a term) about several different things.[381] Before endorsing a substance as a human carcinogen, Professor Furst sought several *valid* studies of humans plus
valid studies in experimental animals at the same exposure levels as
humans that converge to the same conclusion. (Special considerations must be satisfied for "valid" studies of each kind, but I do not

pursue this complex idea.[382]) A variety of other tests would also be needed. As long as one major line of evidence did not clearly converge with others, he would withhold the judgment that the chemical "is a human carcinogen."

(The idea of "ideal" science may also be implicit in strategies that seek to cast doubt on studies. If there is some "doubt" about a body of evidence, interested parties might well argue that this falls short the ideal needed to find a substance toxic (chapter 1).)

In his view, a serious mistake is to judge a substance as a carcinogen when some of his necessary evidence is missing. In contrast, he risks not concluding (or being "dumb") that a substance is a carcinogen, when a substantial, but not ideal, body of evidence shows it is (a scientific false negative). In any case the idea that a mere scintilla of doubt about the toxicity of a substance should not bar public health protections. An opposite mistake would be to require so little evidence that some substances would be judged as carcinogens, when a more robust body of data would show that they were not (scientific false positives).

One could also be "dumb" (but quite concerned) about whether unevaluated chemical creations are carcinogenic to humans simply because public health agencies have not yet assessed them. Demanding copious and highly certain data about each substance in the queue precludes quicker assessment of that product and quicker evaluation of others in commerce but not evaluated, leaving the public ignorant about a large universe of substances and at risk for any that are toxic. In earlier work I argued for expediting aspects of carcinogenic risk assessments so that more toxicants could be assessed in the same amount of time.[383] I briefly reference some of this later in the chapter.

There are also important practical consequences of Furst's ideal. To the extent that certain lines of evidence must be *necessary conditions for inferring toxicity,* this leaves overall assessments about particular substances in limbo.

SOME LIMITATIONS OF EPIDEMIOLOGICAL STUDIES

Using human statistical studies seems especially apt for identifying human toxicants because people are the subjects we wish to protect, but this evidence has substantial limitations. There are also other ways to identify potential adverse effects.

Insensitivity: Some well-known limitations undermine the necessity of epidemiological studies for toxicity assessments. Sample sizes can be too small and statistically underpowered to reliably detect a risk even if it is present. This can easily result in a mistaken "no effect" or false negative result; namely, that there is no evidence that exposure causes an adverse effect. For instance, benzene exposure clearly causes acute promyelocytic leukemia (APL), the disease that afflicted Mr. Milward. However, an epidemiological study would infrequently detect it because it is quite rare. At the time of his trial there were no human studies showing benzene could cause APL. Yet, scientists are highly certain this is true, not on the basis of epidemiological studies, but on other lines of evidence that converge to that conclusion (I return to this below).

The chromium industry, discussed in chapter 1, reduced the statistical power of its initial study by dividing it into two, which ensured that the resulting studies would detect fewer risks and not detect low exposure risks, likely resulting in false negative outcomes.

More generally, epidemiological studies "are not sufficiently sensitive to identify a carcinogenic hazard [or other hazards] except when the risk is high or involves an unusual form of cancer."[384] This is true for very common diseases, such as breast or prostate cancers (it's difficult to separate one cause of these common cancers from another), or quite rare diseases, such as APL. Both public health agencies and tort law judges should ensure that epidemiological studies have low odds of being falsely negative so that toxic effects are not missed.

Not allowing for latency periods: Human studies can be conducted too soon after exposure to reveal a risk. For instance, the latency period between exposure to asbestos and the appearance of mesothelioma is 40 or more years.[385] Consequently, studies conducted 20 or 25 years after exposure might find few or no cases of the disease. Yet, "all forms of asbestos cause mesothelioma and cancers of the lung, larynx and ovary," according to the International Agency for Research on Cancer (IARC).[386]

Similarly, females' in utero exposures to diethylstilbestrol (DES) can result in cervical/vaginal cancer after about a 20-year latency period. Epidemiological studies conducted before the latency period had elapsed might not detect the disease at all or might detect many fewer cases than the exposure might ultimately cause. Thus, researchers must allow sufficient time after exposure to reveal a plausible range of the diseases.

Moreover, when there are long latency periods for diseases— cancers are a prime example—this poses another and serious public health problem: "[Y]ears of preventable human exposures and likely cases of cancer would occur before epidemiological studies could be adequately conducted"[387] and improved health protections could be instituted.

Insufficient understanding of a toxicant: Sometimes there is "insufficient human experience with the agent to determine its full toxicological potential."[388] The toxicity of lead illustrates this. The Greeks and Romans knew lead could cause mental derangement and death. Tetraethyl lead was known as toxic shortly after it was manufactured for gasoline in the 1920s.[389] However, scientists have only recently revealed some of lead's subtle effects in contributing to impulsive and ultimately antisocial behavior.[390]

Crude exposure estimates: Often, exposure assessments for epidemiological studies are "crude and retrospective," undermining accurate results and creating misgivings about the outcome.[391] Yet waiting until there are excellent exposure data circumstances could fail to protect the public if a substance is toxic, especially when there are other ways to determine toxicity.

What do these points reveal about Professor Furst's scientific ideal? If human epidemiological data were *required*, scientifically or legally, to identify a disease, this would likely prevent better health protections and redress in torts. Insisting on a particular kind of evidence that can be quite difficult to obtain will condemn exposed workers or the public to years of preventable diseases and injustices or frustrate redress when they have been harmed.

Demanding epidemiological evidence can also lead to deemphasizing other good evidence. This is particularly important when *other patterns of scientific evidence* are sufficient to reveal human harm, as I consider below.

Studies of humans are attractive because they can provide direct evidence of adverse effects in humans. On some occasions they can identify causal relationships with certainty, even though scientists do not understand the processes by which the adverse effects are produced.[392] However, the limitations just discussed should bar their use as necessary conditions for judgments about human toxicity.

Correctives: Distinguished scientific committees have approaches different from Furst's. Some substances have been identified as known or probable human carcinogens by the IARC or the

US National Toxicology Program (NTP) without good human-statistical data.[393] Some known human carcinogens (several with quite unpronounceable and forgettable names) lack such data: an anticancer drug, 1-(2-chloroethyl)-3-cyclohexyl-1-nitrosourea ("CCNU"); neutron radiation; a substance used in the plastics industry, 4,4'-methylenebis (2-chloroaniline) ("MOCA"); and some benzidine-based dyes that threaten workers.[394] IARC scientists recently identified eight other known human carcinogens without having good human epidemiological data.[395]

However, these few substances are hardly isolated examples. IARC has identified 108 known human carcinogens and also lists 64 substances or groups of substances as *probable human carcinogens*. Importantly, IARC regards both categories of substances as *"equally compelling cancer hazard[s]*; IARC's classification system simply distinguishes whether the data on which that conclusion is based include strong evidence in exposed humans" (emphasis added).[396]

For some of the known human carcinogens, there is little or no statistical human evidence. A total of 35 of the 64 probable human carcinogens have *no human epidemiological data* at all. For the vast majority, the overall classification is based on sufficient evidence in animal studies complemented by "mechanistic and other relevant data," typically genetic or chromosomal damage in animals and sometimes similar damage in cultured human or nonhuman cells.[397]

ANIMAL STUDIES

Furst also requires the use of studies in experimental animals to complement human data. Utilizing animal data is commendable. Distinguished national and international scientific committees concur that animal studies can be importantly relevant for assessing substances that can harm humans.

They have "a complementary set of strengths and limitations" compared with epidemiological studies.[398] That is, they can be good evidence when human data is not or when human studies are less accurate than animal data. They are genuine experiments, exposure is clearly defined and controlled, and experimental conditions can be carefully administered to explore the toxicity of a substance. Typically, they are randomized experiments, with groups of exposed and control animals as the test subjects. Exposed animals are typically dosed with high, medium, and low concentrations of a substance to determine if it *is* toxic and, if so, *how* toxic, at various concentrations.

If statistical tests show greater disease rates in one or more exposed groups compared with the controls, researchers must then determine what the response rates might be in humans by inferring from higher dose outcomes in animals to low-dose effects in humans in order to estimate the toxicity of the substance in humans at typical exposures.[399] Because of the extrapolations, "the question of relevance [to human carcinogenesis or other adverse effects] must be addressed."[400] As one might expect, such inferences are frequently challenged and then strongly denigrated if they threaten corporate interests, but scientists and public health agencies have substantial understanding about how to obtain defensible conclusions for humans.

Strengths: Experimental animal studies have a number of strengths beyond being genuine experiments. First, we should not forget—humans are animals! There are substantial similarities between experimental mammals and humans. Despite some obvious differences between humans and animals that often are emphasized for talking-point, political, regulatory, or litigation purposes when companies are defending products, there are overwhelming similarities. For carcinogens, empirical data "certainly suggests that there are more physiologic, biochemical, and metabolic similarities between laboratory animals and humans than there are differences."[401] Moreover, "biological processes of molecular, cellular, tissue, and organ functions that control life are strikingly similar from one mammalian species to another. [Numerous biological] processes ... vary little in the aggregate as one moves along the phylogenetic ladder."[402]

Second, while there are some differences between animals and humans—humans have longer life spans, may have differential exposures, may process toxicants somewhat differently, and are more heterogeneous—animal studies provide good biological models.[403]

> The similarity in cellular and organ function is particularly strong among mammals such that extrapolation of effects from one species to another is accepted by the scientific community as a means of evaluating the toxicity of external agents.... [T]he specificity of toxic effects on organs is relatively similar across mammals, e.g., a kidney poison in one species is likely to be a kidney poison in another, although there are certainly exceptions. As extrapolation of dose-response from animals to humans is central to deciding appropriate regulatory protection, there is a wealth of research data focusing upon these pathways ... [that] permit[s] reliable extrapolation in many situations.[404]

Consequently, animal studies can provide good evidence for toxicity. Researchers can study and manipulate chemical agents in controlled conditions to identify either beneficial outcomes (e.g., of a pharmaceutical) or harmful effects (e.g., of any number of substances) for humans so that the chemicals are better understood.[405]

Shortcomings: Occasionally, adverse effects in animals may not predict similar results in humans; thus, animal data need to be assessed for what they can and do show about toxic consequences in humans (a point to which Furst was sensitive). For instance, carcinogenic studies typically use high doses and evaluate large numbers of tissues, and some animal strains are prone to high incidences of spontaneous tumors that could be misleading.[406] Yet good scientists understand these limitations, and such studies could be directly germane to workers, particularly susceptible individuals or those who have been subject to accidental exposures. In extremely rare instances an occasional chemical agent may induce tumors in animals through mechanisms that do not operate in humans.[407]

Despite these issues, "it is biologically plausible that agents for which there is *sufficient evidence of carcinogenicity* in experimental animals [IARC's most certain finding] . . . also present a carcinogenic hazard to humans. Accordingly, in the absence of additional scientific information, these agents are considered to pose a carcinogenic hazard to humans."[408]

The importance of animal data: A variety of distinguished scientific committees employ animal data for identifying substances that are toxic to humans: the IARC,[409] the National Academy of Sciences,[410] distinguished scientists from the NTP,[411] California's Proposition 65 Carcinogen Identification Committee,[412] and an independent group of distinguished scientists from major institutions.[413] The Institute of Medicine (IOM) and the National Research Council (NRC) point out their scientific power:

> Animal studies are especially useful in detecting effects of chronic exposures and effects on reproductive and developmental processes because epidemiological methods of studying

humans are especially problematic in these areas.... When well-designed and well-conducted animal studies show adverse effects they should be treated as if similar adverse effects would occur in at least some members of the human population, assuming humans receive a sufficiently high dose.[414]

In spite of their scientific relevance and value, animal studies may be denigrated or maligned by companies with vested interests because this can create doubt about the scientific basis for protecting the public. If companies can convince public health agencies (or tort law judges) to disregard animal data and to use human evidence exclusively, this may well add to the time their products can stay in the market, and definitive results may be more difficult to obtain.[415] And, of course, humans must first be harmed in order to have a record of their health problems show up in epidemiological studies.

Professor Furst endorses animal studies as a necessary condition of certifying that a substance is a human carcinogen. However, a few known human carcinogens initially did not cause tumors in animals.[416] Thus, if animal data were regarded as a *necessary condition* for inferring toxic effects in humans, their absence would preclude the judgment that a substance is toxic for mistaken reasons.

Despite many virtues, animal studies have some limitations for pubic health purposes. They are not quick experiments, taking five to seven years to conduct and interpret and requiring many person-hours of effort to carry out. They are also expensive. Ideally, scientists need to find quicker, short-term tests to reliably identify toxicants. In addition, animal experiments have unfortunately declined at least in part because of concerns about proper treatment of the animals.

OTHER EVIDENCE ASSISTS
THE IDENTIFICATION OF TOXICANTS

Mechanistic studies—data that reveal key biological steps in pathways leading to adverse effects—can be quite powerful evidence. For cancers, mechanistic studies include "data on pre-neoplastic lesions, tumor pathology, genetic and related effects, structure–activity relationships, metabolism and toxicokinetics, physicochemical parameters and analogous biological agents."[417] These "pivotal data" have become more prominent recently for identifying toxicants, importantly supporting the classification of substances as "known" or "probable" human carcinogens when human statistical data are not conclusive (or absent)[418] and quite rarely, downgrading chemicals to less toxic classifications.

The IARC recognizes a trade-off between human statistical data and "the strength of the mechanistic data needed . . ."[419] Mechanistic evidence can substitute "for conventional epidemiological studies when there is less than sufficient evidence in humans," when it shows that a substance has biological effects in humans similar to those in animals.[420] It can also "substitute for conventional cancer [animal] bioassays when there is less than sufficient evidence in experimental animals."[421]

As noted above, IARC upgraded 6 agents to "known human carcinogens" and 38 to probable human carcinogens, using mechanistic evidence.[422] Thus, 38 substances, which previously would not have been considered as carcinogens, are now understood as cancerous compounds from which the public should be protected.

However, biological mechanisms often may not be known. Consequently, if such evidence is *demanded* as a necessary condition, as it occasionally has been by some tort law judges (more below), waiting for it could slow scientific and legally authoritative findings and continue ignorance as well as harm and injustice to those exposed. For instance, the mechanisms of aspirin's benefits and harms were not understood for more than 100 years.[423] Also, currently there is little or no mechanistic understanding of how statins cause muscle damage and thalidomide causes shortened limbs. "The history of science is replete with solid causal conclusions in advance of solid mechanistic understanding," according to a National Academy of Sciences committee.[424]

Manufacturers strategically try to defend their products by pressuring public health agencies to have extensive bodies of data (resembling Furst's suggestions), myriad levels of scientific review, and high degrees of certainty (no "doubt") before the public is better protected. Despite companies' sometimes dishonorable approaches toward science, their hired experts may portray themselves as scientific angels, arguing that the very "best and most certain" science must support legal actions. They then argue that departures from this ideal because of "insufficient" data, no data of certain kinds, or an insufficiently complete "data set" generate "enough doubt" that no legal action should be taken to safeguard the public. If public health agencies succumb to such arguments or if administrative procedures require them to consider such data, this will preclude timely health protections (as we saw in chapter 1). In effect, companies would succeed in creating toxic ignorance ("without the best science, we don't yet know enough") and slow authoritative assessments of toxicity, sacrifice public health protections, lead to more-adverse effects, and continue existing injustices against citizens.

A POSTMARKET ALTERNATIVE
TO FURST'S IDEAL

When public health agencies assess the toxicity of substances in commerce, they should utilize and integrate all the varieties of scientific evidence relevant to toxicity assessments. There should be no necessary kind of data as Furst urged.

There should be no hierarchy of evidence for toxicity and no necessarily required kinds of evidence, according to the National Cancer Institute.[425] A National Academy of Sciences committee has endorsed a similar point, as if responding to Furst: "It seems impossible and undesirable to build a scientifically defensible framework in which evidence is integrated in a completely explicit, fixed, and predefined recipe or algorithm."[426]

Sometimes there will be good human studies, sometimes not. Sometimes there will be good animal data and few or no human data. Sometimes good mechanistic data is available that can serve instead of animal or human data, and so on. Researchers and agencies should consider the total body of scientifically relevant evidence that is readily available to determine how it does or does not "fit together" to credibly assess the toxicity of a chemical creation. If missing data are needed to complete the scientific picture, they should seek it out or develop it. (Also, to the extent it is legally possible public health agencies should not automatically accept new human data just because they are "statistically significant." They should ensure that the studies have sufficient statistical power (low false negative rates) to identify risks, if they are present.) However, they should free themselves from a priori and necessary kinds of evidence in order to better and more quickly assess toxicants to protect the public. Indeed, these are current policies at research agencies such as the IARC and the NTP, along with regulatory agencies such as the US and the California Environmental Protection Agencies (EPAs).[427]

Unfortunately, the EPA is under substantial political and other pressures to employ human data and to have multiple studies of various kinds, creating a database that likely constitutes excessive science. Moreover, the lack of funding and personnel hamstrings its efforts. However, scientific overkill policies are likely to stymie timely public health actions, to result in more diseases and dysfunctions, and to kill more citizens.

Finally, because scientific studies march to their own usually slow cadence and depend on the availability of evidence, the more kinds of data that are needed for toxicity assessments, the more problems this poses. Efforts to prudently protect the public must take into account the typical duration of scientific studies and when possible shorten this duration or find quicker alternatives to provide the needed data under postmarket laws.

IMPROVING POSTMARKET SCIENCE

In the current legal environment even with the Lautenberg Act becoming law, postmarket actions to reduce toxic risks will continue to be a fact of life. While the Lautenberg Act has changed aspects of the legal landscape and introduced some important correctives to the 1976 TSCA, substantial shortcomings remain. Consider some important legal features that in principle address several shortcomings of the 1976 TSCA.

1) The EPA "must make an affirmative finding on the safety of a new chemical or significant new use of an existing chemical before it is allowed into the marketplace."[428] It must "consider

risks to susceptible and highly exposed populations [these may include infants, pregnant women, children and workers] and ensure a substance does not pose an "unreasonable risk." This is a major improvement. In order for it to function well, the agency must hold proposed new substances to good evidentiary standards and careful review to protect the public. How well EPA does this will be revealed as it implements the law. Of course, at the moment no product has been reviewed under the new procedures.

2) If needed evidence is missing, the EPA can more easily demand it by an *administrative order* rather than using a time-consuming notice and rule-making[429], which in the past could take three years. No specific toxicity tests appear to be required for identifying toxic effects, as there are for pharmaceuticals and pesticides. This appears to give EPA flexibility to decide on what kinds and amounts of data it needs for particular substances, but it may also open the door for companies to pressure the agency not to require some data. If this premarket provision functions well, it would reduce legal battery from new substances (Chapter 2).

Statutory language encourages the EPA to find substitutes for animal studies, if they are available. However, such data is among the best non-human studies for assessing the toxicity of a product. (Also, sufficiently accurate surrogates may not be easily found.) It thus moves in the direction of "no data, no market."[430] However, EPA must strongly commit to enforcing this last provision.

3) The amendments mandate safety reviews for all chemicals currently in "active commerce," namely those a company has manufactured in the last ten years. Within the first six months after the date of enactment the EPA must have 10 ongoing

risk evaluations and must have "20 ongoing risk evaluations within 3.5 years."[431] Another 20 substances may be requested by manufacturers for the EPA to review. Surprisingly, only twenty of the 40 total need be "high priorities" from a health and environmental perspective.[432]

4) Existing substances pose a substantial problem because the 1976 TSCA permitted 84,000 substances into commerce with little understanding of their toxicity and no magic wand will quickly update their toxicity data. As few as 30,000 of these products may be "active" in commerce (the actual number is unknown). However, even if the EPA could successfully and completely review the toxicity of 20 *each* year, an unheard of rapid rate, it would still take 1500 years to review just the "active" substances about most of which we are ignorant. If EPA takes *seven years* for each twenty substances, this will reduce the pace of evaluation to that of a snail. Not all commercial chemicals will pose risks, but EPA must review plausible candidates and then evaluate a subset of them in depth. A major risk is, "that the agency we have today will soon become mired in 'paralysis by analysis' before it takes action and a flood of litigation after it–only occasionally–acts."[433] California state officials who know the workings of EPA intimately have similar concerns. However, might "doing risk assessment and regulation correctly" but slowly, send an important message to manufacturers to remove risky product from the market before they face legal review? Nonetheless, the EPA must attend to greater efficiency in reviewing products to better protect the public.

Concerns raised earlier in the book about the legacy of untested products will plague postmarket evaluations of products, but it should be easier for EPA to obtain data about products under review. Nonetheless, the EPA could well be overwhelmed in implementing the Lautenberg Act. (We should note that even as risks from high priority products are reduced and fewer people put at risk or harmed, "residual" harms to the public may still continue simply because of earlier exposures.)

5) EPA must give priority to chemicals that are persistent, bio-accumulative, and are known human carcinogens or otherwise have high toxicity. This is an important addition.

6) The costs of reviewing new and existing chemicals is a concern. Although industry must contribute (up to) $25 million per year toward myriad reviewing activities, this amount is likely inadequate, given EPA's increased responsibilities for a large body of substances. It is also woefully small given industry's touted annual income of $800 billion. Even manufacturers' annual contributions can be put at risk if congress fails to fund EPA at a sufficient level.[434]

7) In implementing these reviews, there are aggressive and judicially enforceable deadlines for EPA actions that many commentators applaud.[435] These likely will face considerable litigation and other pressures and possibly be eroded over time. Public and administrative support for EPA's efforts might help counterbalance manufacturers' efforts to slow health protections.

8) Costs may not be considered when EPA conducts risk analyses, an improvement compared with the 1976 TSCA. However, EPA must determine the "reasonably ascertainable economic consequences of a protective *regulation*, including its 'likely effect on the *national economy*,' phrasing that parrots the worst language of existing law" (emphasis added).[436] Because one cost-benefit analysis can be hundreds of pages long, this could greatly slow efforts to protect the public.

9) The Lautenberg Act preserves some state authority and laws that have protected the American public from toxicants when federal laws failed, but it decreases other state actions.[437] Important long-standing laws in California and Massachusetts, *inter alia,* appear to be exempt. However, once EPA issues a final health standard for a substance, state laws must be consistent with that; they cannot be more protective, contrary to other federal-state interactions. States may institute better protections if federal protections are too slow.

10) Because of the preceding issues, a little noticed point is that reducing states' power to protect the pubic permits industry to concentrate its lobbying influence at the federal EPA, where past practice suggests it will likely seek to slow protective standards without having to modify their products to meet state regulations. The public's health might not be well protected.

11) The public appears to be poorly protected from imported products from countries with less protective laws, e.g., lead in children's jewelry, or phthalates or BPA in other products.

12) Confidential business information exemptions will be somewhat more difficult to use, likely increasing some information about substances to which the public is exposed.[438]

13) If a chemical has been phased out, such as C8, a toxicologically unknown replacement should not be able to go into production under the new law. Instead this should trigger a "new use" or "greater production" assessment of the product. EPA then should be able to make a safety determination about it with appropriate data. This would be a substantial improvement. Had the Lautenberg Act been in effect when DuPont tried to introduce shorter chain variants of C8, these should have been subject to a safety review. In fact

DuPont has already introduced such products, with little known about them, and researchers are already concerned about their toxicity.

MOVING FORWARD UNDER THE LAUTENBERG ACT WITH IMPROVING SCIENCE

Addressing existing chemicals in commerce approved under the 1976 TSCA will essentially require toxicity assessments of unknown substances under postmarket circumstances that entered commerce under that law. It will be easier for EPA to demand data than earlier. In addition to demanding data from manufacturers what else could be done? Could there be scientific progress that would reduce exposures, some injustices, and misery? Could various kinds of "scouting" help identify chemically burdened populations and likely toxicants earlier? We now consider some possibilities.

SCOUTING FOR HEIGHTENED EXPOSURES

Currently, the Biomonitoring Program of the Centers for Disease Control and Prevention (CDC) and some states, such as California, scout for elevated community or workplace exposures to toxicants. With reliable protocols for detecting toxicants in blood and urine, biomonitoring can discover concentrations of suspected toxicants in the general population and people at greater risk.

California's Biomonitoring Program has gone further, seeking to detect elevated concentrations of toxicants in targeted subpopulations such as firefighters, people living near toxic waste dumps, pregnant women, teenagers who use copious amounts of cosmetics, and farmworkers.[439] Some health agencies routinely sample breast milk for toxicants during this especially vulnerable period of developing children's lives.

Scouting for cumulative impacts would importantly expand biomonitoring. This should include people who are exposed to multiple toxicants because of where they work, the homes they live in, or where they live.[440]

SCOUTING FOR DISEASES

Once health agencies found heightened contamination from toxicants, they could target those subpopulations in order to identify any diseases as early as is clinically possible. This would likely be too late to prevent some illnesses but it might help identify people for early intervention and medical assistance if they needed it.[441]

ACCELERATING TOXICITY DATA

In order to expedite health protections, agencies could incorporate toxicity findings from other credible and authoritative bodies. This would avoid reinventing the toxicological results already in the literature. For instance, California's Proposition 65 cancer and reproductive science advisory panels incorporate the findings of IARC, the NTP, the US Food and Drug Administration (FDA), the EPA, and the National Institute of Occupational Safety and Health (NIOSH) to identify toxicants.[442] Thus, shortly after IARC concluded that the herbicide Roundup was a probable human carcinogen, California listed it as a carcinogen.

In addition, some features about chemical agents or their metabolites potentially can provide early clues to toxicity. Persistent and bioaccumulating substances should be scrutinized as scientists are doing and the Lautenberg Act requires. Persistent substances remain in the environment and typically in human bodies for longer periods of time, providing multiple opportunities for exposure. PCBs have half-lives in humans of about eight years, while the polybrominated flame retardants (PBDEs) and C8 have half-lives of two to three years.[443] Some substances, such as PCBs, increase in toxicity as they move up the food chain. Some bioaccumulate (build up) in human (and other mammalian) bodies, increasing internal doses.

Scientists were alerted to concerns about PBDEs because they had concentrated in birds of prey. PBDEs chemically resemble PCBs, known toxicants, which suggested similar biological consequences for people, indicated the need for study, and increased the importance of the alert.[444] As a result, researchers urged the public health community to focus attention on the PBDEs.

Some substances act by similar mechanisms or bind to certain cellular receptors, having common toxic effects. This is true of so-called dioxin-like compounds and organophosphate pesticides (see chapter 2).[445] Researchers could also seek others; this is occurring for endocrine disrupters. Sometimes the search for similar compounds, such as endocrine disrupters, also reveals similar diseases as occurred recently with DDT (chapter 2).

"UPSTREAM" SEARCHES FOR TOXICANTS

Researchers are beginning to search for precursors of adverse effects "upstream" from actual clinical diseases. They could look for substances that affect the same biological endpoints that lead to disease. For instance, dioxin-like PCBs, non-dioxin-like PCBs, perchlorate, and PBDEs operating via different biological pathways can reduce thyroid concentrations in pregnant women, threatening children's neurological development (see chapter 2).[446] If scientists could make identification of these pathways sufficiently precise, we would not have to wait for diseases to appear.

Toxicants can also be identified earlier by their mechanisms of biological action. For instance, an NTP scientist, Ron Melnick, identified 12 high-volume, epoxide-forming chemicals that produce mutagens and likely cause cancer. Seven were known human carcinogens (e.g., vinyl chloride, ethylene oxide, benzene) or probable human carcinogens (e.g., vinyl bromide, vinyl fluoride, styrene oxide, glycidol). However, five had been ignored by public health agencies because they were merely classified as "possible" human carcinogens or not classified at all. Yet, all act by a common mechanism, likely posing hazards to humans and making them live threats. Chemical and mechanistic considerations provide substantial insights for identifying less well-studied substances as harmful.[447] Subsequently, IARC upgraded styrene, vinyl bromide, and vinyl fluoride on the basis of the kinds of considerations that Melnick urged.[448] And IARC has generalized the use of mechanistic data to good effect.

As this book goes to press, a large team of scientists has embarked on "the Next Generation (NexGen) of Risk Assessment."[449] This is a more recent generalization of some of the ideas above: more-rapid identification of chemicals of concern, more precise characterization of "mechanisms of action that influence conclusions about causality," and "[elucidation of] new biomarkers of exposure and effects."[450]

MINING EXISTING KNOWLEDGE

The suggestions above urge the mining of existing knowledge to anticipate new risks. Researchers might seek "susceptibility genes," while others might seek deep biological analogies to reveal unexpected toxic properties.[451] Still others, using a simple test for mutagenicity, have found that 20% of the created chemical universe, including high-production chemicals, is mutagenic, damaging DNA.[452] This test could have identified mutagens before they entered commerce, or could now be used to determine whether high-exposure or other substances are mutagens.

EXPEDITING TOXICITY ASSESSMENTS

Some steps in postmarket risk assessment can be expedited, as some of us illustrated in the mid-1990s. Previously, carcinogenic potency assessments had taken one-half to five person-years per substance. This was science intensive, labor intensive, costly, and slow. Our procedures produced accurate potencies for carcinogens at a rate of about one chemical per day, provided that appropriate animal data were available.[453] This is 1/365th of a person-year, compared to earlier rates.[454]

It appears far better to review and assess a large number of substances (even with occasional differences from long, slow estimates) than to leave a substantial universe of substances unassessed and the public at risk. The California EPA adopted these procedures into law under Proposition 65.[455]

Finally, authoritative "substances-of-concern" lists could alert citizens to potential toxicants and might encourage firms to change products or processes.[456] Proposition 65 lists carcinogens and reproductive toxicants that the public or health agencies can be utilized as a guide to toxicity.[457]

LIMITATIONS OF SUGGESTED "IMPROVEMENTS"

At this time, almost none of the ideas just suggested would actually reduce exposures or reduce diseases. Some come closer than others: a public health agency incorporating toxicity data from other agencies, analogues to Melnick's recommendations, and the NexGen risk assessment perhaps come closest, but even these require further implementation. The strategies, such as biomonitoring and Proposition 65-type lists, provide early warnings about potential disease-causing exposures or identify highly exposed subpopulations or perhaps diseases in certain communities. Some accelerate critical knowledge steps in the regulatory process by means of precursors of diseases or known toxic mechanisms. All help, but there are limitations to each.

Together they can help authoritatively publicize the toxicity of products and assist some public health protections, but because some of the ideas amount to (accurately) estimating toxicity or potency of exposures, they could remain open to challenge by industries' "scientific angels" because they do not identify diseases in actual people. If public health agencies are so pressured, what will they do?

When science is used well after exposures have occurred and after diseases may have been triggered, public health agencies should utilize some of the second-best suggestions to expeditiously reduce hazards and unjust treatment of citizens as best they can.

The best science-law public health solution

The best approach to protecting the public from chemical creations and preventing ignorance and injustice is to implement a variation of premarket toxicity testing. This would allow scientific studies to identify most toxicants before they enter the public sphere, pose risks and cause harm. I have presented this point elsewhere.[458]

Congress has now moved in this direction. It has also sought to have some legally mandated procedures so that the toxicity of existing products can proceed quicker. Several National Academy of Sciences committees in endorsing similar proposals[459] suggest that the testing must be implemented in a practical manner that protects the public health. For instance, "the intensity and depth of testing should be based on practical needs, including the use of the chemical, the likelihood of human exposure, and the scientific questions that such testing must answer to support a reasonable science-policy decision."[460] One committee notes, "It is neither practical nor desirable to attempt to test every chemical (or mixture) against every end point during a wide range of life stages . . . A well-designed tiered strategy could help to set priorities among environmental agents for screening and could identify end points of mechanisms of action that would trigger more in-depth testing for various end points or in various life stages."[461]

Some benefits of premarket testing: Premarket toxicity testing under the Lautenberg Act going forward can be quite accurate if agencies choose appropriate individual studies within a reasonable range of accuracy and a reasonable range of costs. Such tests would also better serve justice and would remove many concerns about legal battery because fewer people would be exposed to substances of unknown toxicity.[462]

An appropriate array of tests would ensure fewer short-term and minor harms in violation of John Rawls's first principle of justice. Tests could additionally identify quite serious effects on the neurological, reproductive, and immune systems, among others, screening out toxic products that would undermine or truncate citizens' lifetime opportunities. These might include heavy-metal poisoning, childhood cancer, serious asthma, intellectual disability, autism, attention deficit disorder, breast and prostate cancers, and Parkinson's disease, inter alia. Premarket testing might have reduced the risks and harms to Jeromy Darling, Ken Wamsley, Carla Bartlett, and Sandy Guest, if it had been in place earlier.

If testing reduces adverse effects for those in lower socioeconomic groups who work in chemical-intensive industries, work on farms, or live in areas heavily contaminated by toxicants, this would diminish some of the current effects that exacerbate inequalities of income and wealth.[463]

The social efficacy of premarket testing: From an impartial social point of view economic studies suggest that premarket toxicity testing of chemical creations would be quite efficient and a bargain compared with the costs of childhood disease attributable to chemical exposures.[464] In Europe under REACH, the 11-year cost to test and review 30,000 chemicals is less than one euro per European citizen per year for 11 years, or about $5 billion total.[465]

For comparison, the *one-year* costs of childhood diseases alone in 2008 from lead poisoning, asthma, intellectual disability, autism, attention deficit disorder, and childhood cancers were approximately $76.6 billion.[466] Thus, to the extent that the above estimates provide reasonable guidance, there is an overwhelming case for premarket toxicity testing for chemical creations that can contribute to such diseases. Even if a few toxicants are missed in the process, the data suggest that the costs to reduce *only* childhood diseases (ignoring all others) would be quite reasonable.

From the industry point of view, concerns about costs also appear less worrisome than companies might argue. A study for the Norwegian Council of Ministers estimating the costs to implement the REACH legislation in Europe found that testing 30,000 substances might increase the costs of chemical products by 0.063 of 1 percent at the low end to 0.20 of 1 percent at the high end. For contrast, the spot price of oil changes this much 51 out of 52 weeks per year, hardly a radical price variation.[467] Consequently, if a chemical costs 100,000 euros per barrel (an invented number) before testing, an increase of 0.20 of 1 percent (the higher number) would increase the sale price to 100,200 euros per barrel over 11 years. An extra 200 euros per barrel is not likely to adversely affect social resources, bankrupt individual companies, or put downstream users out of business.[468]

Total costs of testing the 30,000 substances under REACH over the 11-year phase-in are a tiny fraction of the chemical industry's profits. In 2003 the *annual* revenues of the European chemical industry were 356 billion euros, or 100 times greater than the estimated 11-year testing costs. Over an 11-year period in constant dollars, total industry income would be about 3.916 trillion euros. These estimates would be about 0.089 of 1 percent of total revenues for 1 year. Even if the high-end testing costs were several times higher, they seem quite reasonable.[469]

Premarket testing for the toxic properties of chemical creations, required by justice, seems efficient in relative to the current circumstances.

HOW SCIENCE REQUIREMENTS IN THE TORT LAW CAN FRUSTRATE THE POSSIBILITY OF REDRESS

When some citizens have been harmed by chemical exposures, they can seek redress in the tort law. When they do, they will need to present scientific evidence in that legal venue. How should scientific issues in the tort law be addressed in court cases to bettr ensure plaintiffs receive just treatment?

The pressures that can frustsrate redress of harm in a tort case come both from defendants and some judges. Defendants seek to persuade judges that they should demand certain kinds of evidence before plaintiffs' experts are permitted to present scientific testimony to a jury. Judges' decisions or those required by appellate precedents might result in similar views (recall Mr. Milward's district court fate). Thus, judicial choices are quite important in adjudicating the science needed for tort law adjudication.

On the one hand, courts can require "too much" or "too little" science in support of testimony. On the other hand, they can more appropriately follow the Supreme Court's guidance that recognizes testimony should go to a jury when reasonable scientists would disagree, "even though the evidence is 'shaky.'"[470]

What I briefly describe below as "mistakes" by judges resemble several problems just rehearsed for public health agencies, so the discussion is shorter. However, the errors in tort cases can vary by trial courts or by appellate jurisdictions because of their decentralization. There can also be more numerous and more visible errors from court decisions because judges, not trained in science, are buffeted by adversarial experts but do not have knowledgeable support from informed scientists to guide them as do health agencies.

In summary, some courts have insisted that experts must have certain kinds of evidence that are good or desirable but not scientifically necessary to draw conclusions about toxic effects in humans. At other times they mistakenly excluded relevant evidence that scientists normally use to infer the toxicity of substances.[471] Both can adversely and unnecessarily constrain expert testimony and frustrate justice. Courts have also had difficulty understanding the nature of scientific reasoning (see chapter 3).[472] Consider each of these in brief.

DEMANDS FOR IDEAL EVIDENCE

Some judicial rulings shortly after the *Daubert* decision demanded "textbook evidence" resembling Furst's ideal. A district court in the *Wade-Greaux* case, adjudicating whether a mother's use of Primatene Tablets and Primatene Mist "caused TiaNicole Wade-Greaux to be born with true malformation of her upper limbs and other skeletal defects,"[473] placed exacting restrictions on expert testimony.[474] It required the plaintiffs to support their case by "repeated, consistent epidemiological studies; an animal model that duplicates the defects resulting in the human from the exposure; a dose/response relationship between the exposure and the effect on the experimental fetus; and . . . the mechanism of teratogenicity of the agent should be understood and make biologic sense."[475]

The trial judge prohibited the plaintiffs' testimony because some of the evidence was missing, and the Third Circuit Court of Appeals upheld it.[476] Was the proposed support for testimony necessarily inadequate? Could there have been a less than ideal evidence to support the testimony? I do not know, but one observation seems clear. If limb malformations are rare and the use of Primatene Mist during pregnancy is sufficiently rare, human studies may not be able to detect risks, even if they exist.[477] Demanding such full evidence would prevent almost all cases from going to trial. Yet, other kinds of evidence can be quite sufficient to identify adverse effects and support expert testimony.[478]

While the ruling in this case represents an extreme view of the science needed to support expert testimony and is a mistaken outlier, because it lurks in the history of legal decisions it could mistakenly influence other courts.[479]

MORE SPECIFIC SHORTCOMINGS

Beyond demands for a total body of ideal scientific evidence, some courts have approached this by demanding specific kinds of scientific data to support expert testimony. A common demand is for human epidemiological evidence, a prevalent legacy from the Bendectin cases, which includes *Daubert*.[480] The Texas Supreme Court (not a federal court) has gone much further—a plaintiff at the bar must have at least two human epidemiological studies and the plaintiff's exposures and circumstances must sufficiently resemble people in the studies in order to survive dismissal of his or her case.[481] This would more than double the difficulty of redressing of harms.

Human statistical data can be good evidence of human harm, but we have seen several reasons such evidence may not be available or accurate. However, such studies should not be necessary conditions for testimony, just as they should not be required for public health decisions. Moreover, if courts demand this type of data, this will squeeze out or lead to denigrating other perfectly good studies.[482]

Fixed and low statistical-significance restrictions: Some courts have also imposed *legal* restrictions on epidemiological evidence. For instance, they have insisted that human studies must be "statistically significant at the 0.05 level." That is, the statistical chances of a study mistakenly reporting an adverse effect when there is none (a false positive) should be no greater than 1 chance out of 20. (This is also expressed as a 95% confidence interval.) This would require scientists to accept a "causal claim only if they can show that the odds of the relationship's occurring by chance are no more than one in 20 . . . [however,] if there's more than even a scant 5 percent possibility that an event occurred by chance, scientists" would have to reject the claim.[483]

This legal demand is a problematic decision rule because it increases the chances that the study might fail to detect adverse outcomes even if they are present.[484] It could lead to false-negative mistakes, failing "to protect people who are really getting hurt."[485] The EPA adopted only a slightly higher chance of false positives— 0.10 instead of 0.05—to ensure that it did not miss adverse effects from involuntary smoke exposure, which causes lung cancer. The cigarette industry no doubt objected to the decision, but the public, along with those who serve them in airplanes, restaurants, and bars, is better protected.

Radiation epidemiology illustrates the same point. Atomic-bomb survivors from Hiroshima and Nagasaki contracted leukemias and multiple myeloma, as well as cancer of the esophagus, stomach, urinary tract, lung, lymph nodes, colon, other segments of the digestive system, and other sites.[486]

Epidemiological studies show with (importantly) 90% confidence that all malignant neoplasms taken together (except leukemia) have a relative risk of less than 2.0. Only a few diseases—leukemia, multiple myeloma, urinary tract, and colon cancer—have relative risks greater than 2.0 from radiation exposure.

Importantly, the radiation studies have two properties that some tort judges might use to exclude expert testimony: relative risks for many tumors are less than 2.0 and they were identified with a 90% confidence interval. Yet causation has been established and radiation is widely known for these cancers, which resulted from surprisingly low exposures.

Court-imposed decision rules for low statistical significance rates create another barrier for parties seeking redress for chemical-caused injuries. If courts endorse it, they decide that in the law it is more important to avoid mistakenly condemning a substance as toxic when it is not (which protects defendants) than to miss a toxic effect that could be present (which would better serve injured plaintiffs). The rule also makes decisions less "accurate."[487] Rejecting all studies that are not statistically significant at 0.05 "would be a cursory and foolish judgment, particularly if there are multiple studies tending to show a consistent effect."[488]

This particular requirement is also contrary to how responsible and good scientists conduct their own research. Scientists tolerate a wider range of statistical variation for interpreting studies because they understand how to interpret what the studies show and do not show about the data.

Requiring relative risks greater than 2.0: Numerous other courts have required human studies to show that an exposed group of people has a disease rate that is at least *twice as great* as the disease rate in the general population, or a "relative risk" greater than 2.0. For some courts, if this condition is not satisfied, experts will not be permitted to address juries and plaintiffs' cases will be dismissed.[489]

However, a general causal relation between exposure and disease can be established with certainty with a relative risk less than 2.0 If judges exclude such data, this could preclude testimony about clear causal relations, including radiation-caused cancers. "Involuntary" tobacco smoke can cause lung cancer, yet there is only a 20% elevated rate of lung cancer from the exposure, a relative risk of 1.2. Combined estrogen-progestogen contraception causes breast cancer with a relative risk of 1.3 to 1.43.[490] Those who eat a daily portion of processed meat have an elevated risk of cancer 1.18 times greater than those who do not eat processed meat.[491] In all these instances, causation is certain but the relative risk is small compared to high relative risks from smoking causing lung cancer (relative risk of 10).

There is a cautionary point to be noted. While general causation—that an exposure can cause a disease—can be established with relative risks less than two, a further issue in torts is that a plaintiff must show "specific causation," that his or her exposure more likely than not *did* cause his or her disease. This could be more difficult without a relative risk being greater than two, yet there are other ways to show this by ruling out other plausible causes of a person's disease.[492]

Requiring mechanistic evidence for each step of a disease process: A few courts have imposed other misleading requirements on scientific testimony that could mistakenly keep plaintiffs from even having a chance to redress harms they suffered. One court required plaintiffs to have mechanistic evidence for each step of a disease process in support of expert testimony.[493] While mechanistic data can importantly contribute to toxicity findings, to require information on every mechanistic link from exposure to disease would create a virtually impossible barrier. The plaintiffs were excluded from trial. Such evidence will only rarely, if ever, be available for any causal pathway from exposure to disease.[494]

Denigrating animal data: Many courts have denigrated animal studies or have excluded plaintiffs who sought to rely on them. In an effort to eliminate some plaintiffs' evidence defendants often say "humans are not big rats or mice." If they persuade some courts of this point, these ideas will be difficult to dislodge because of written precedent. In an Agent Orange case, a well-known federal judge held (1) that servicemen and women were not exposed to the high doses of Agent Orange to which experimental animals were exposed, and (2) because the experimental animals were of a different species than humans, the use of these studies would be so "potentially misleading as to be inadmissible."[495] In a Bendectin case, the Fifth Circuit Court of Appeals asserted that animal studies were of "questionable applicability to humans," especially in the absence of some reference to epidemiological studies.[496] This view was echoed in later cases.

Yet this is contrary to scientific research. Scientists routinely use animal data to infer toxic effects in humans. Sometimes animal data alone can decisively identify adverse effects for humans. At other times they are especially powerful, particularly when complemented by information about toxic biological mechanisms. Bernard Goldstein (referenced above at note 403) has quite ably argued for the point that "humans are animals."[497] Legally precluding animal data to support expert testimony will deprive experts of important and relevant data on which scientists routinely rely.

Precluding the use of case reports: Some courts have become so enamored of statistical evidence that they will not permit plaintiffs to use human case reports as part of the database of expert testimony because they lack various statistical features. Case reports usually arise from a concern that two concurrent events, such as a disease and a certain exposure, happen more frequently "than would be expected by chance."[498] Some aspects of courts' concerns are reasonable, as case studies do have shortcomings compared with statistical studies: they typically report single observations, do not comprehensively identify all instances of the same disease in a population or a population at risk, and do not estimate the number of cases of disease when there is no exposure (although sometimes this can be calculated).[499]

Case reports may or may not provide relevant evidence. Some may be *merely descriptive*, reporting, for example, a simple temporal relationship between an exposure and disease; these would be of no scientific relevance. Others, *much more detailed*, are more important and relevant. They might involve *dechallenges*: a person became sick after taking a drug but then no longer took the drug and her health improved. They could be *rechallenges*: the person became sick while using a drug but ceased taking it and improved, then returned to taking it and became sick again.[500] There could be good analyses of potential causes, ruling out explanations that the evidence does not support. Despite some limitations, an IOM-NRC committee points out, "In summary, **higher concern is warranted in situations where one or more well-documented serious adverse events manifest positive temporality, and other factors (e.g., positive dechallenge, biological plausibility, or laboratory results) combine to strengthen the perceived association between the dietary supplement ingested and the adverse event in question**" (bold in original).[501] On the basis of nine human case reports and some mechanistic evidence, the IOM-NRC committee concluded that the dietary supplement chaparral could be toxic to human livers and kidneys.[502]

Similarly, in 1974 occupational physicians and their collaborators reported three cases "of angiosarcoma of the liver among workers at a polyvinyl chloride (PVC) production plant in Louisville."[503] Searches at other plants revealed eight more cases. *No* epidemiological studies at the time were available. On the basis of 11 case reports, animal data, and elevated risks compared with the general population, these scientists concluded that "exposure to VCM [vinyl chloride monomer] in the course of VC polymerization work *is responsible* for malignant and nonmalignant liver" (emphasis added).[504]

IARC routinely considers good case reports as relevant data.[505] It classified MOCA as a known human carcinogen, without human statistical studies. MOCA is a multiorgan carcinogen in animals,[506] and MOCA-caused DNA adducts found in animals were also seen in a few exposed humans. MOCA exhibits obvious genotoxic mechanisms.[507] A scoping technique used in urinary tracts revealed two individuals with early-stage bladder cancer after only brief exposures to MOCA. MOCA *is* a human carcinogen.

Unfortunately, if experts testifying in some trial courts about the toxicity of MOCA had referenced the two case reports showing early-stage bladder cancers, along with the other data but without epidemiological data, they might have been excluded. If experts were unable to testify in court, an injured party with bladder cancer because of exposure to MOCA would have been deprived of the possibility of redress for the harm suffered. The court would not have issued an authoritative ruling that MOCA could cause cancer in other employees. The affected company might not have modified MOCA workplace processes.

Some courts have permitted case reports, but importantly the US Supreme Court recently endorsed them as evidence for causation (in a fraud case), rejecting the idea that "statistical significance is the only reliable indication of causation."[508]

SCIENTIFIC REASONING IN THE TORT LAW

Some courts have peremptorily excluded litigants' weight of the evidence, diagnostic induction, or inference to the best explanation arguments. For instance, the Fifth Circuit Court of Appeal objected to them. It was "unpersuaded that the 'weight of the evidence' methodology . . . is scientifically acceptable for demonstrating [medical causation because. . . . [t]his methodology results from the preventive perspective that the agencies adopt in order to reduce public exposure to harmful substances."[509] The court was simply mistaken in its reasoning.

Distinguished scientific committees assessing the toxic causal processes of substances endorse such inferences. The IARC[510] and NTP[511] explicitly employ a weight of the evidence process that considers numerous lines of evidence and integrates them to reach cause-effect conclusions,. However, the idea that they use lesser scientific standards in their arguments is mistaken. They are particularly cautious scientific organizations that are not too quick to identify carcinogens.

In addition, the form of the argument can support conclusions that satisfy different standards of proof. An inference to the best explanation could be used to infer "beyond a reasonable doubt" that a poison was used to kill a victim in a criminal case.[512] In short, the *form of the argument* is not committed to a particular *standard of proof* to infer the conclusion.

The First Circuit's *Milward* opinion also contrasts the *Allen* case from *Milward*:[513] "No serious argument can be made that the weight of the evidence approach is inherently unreliable. Rather, admissibility must turn on the particular facts of the case."[514]

Individual scientists and investigators utilize a weight of the evidence methodology to arrive at cause-effect relationships and conclusions.[515] This is particularly clear in the biological sciences.[516] Among others, epidemiologists,[517] toxicologists, methodologists inferring causes from well-analyzed case studies,[518] governmental scientists assessing risks, and investigators seeking to explain airplane or space shuttle accidents[519] also employ such inferences.

In inferences to the best explanation, different lines of evidence may play a greater or lesser role in supporting a toxicity judgment, *depending on what other evidence may be available in a particular case.* "Epidemiology, animal, tissue culture and molecular pathology should be seen as integrating evidences in the determination of human carcinogenicity."[520] The inferences organize arguments to conclusions that the data support and guide the integration of evidence. IOM-NRC notes,

> Available evidence from each category of data, by itself may be insufficient to indicate concern [from dietary supplements], but when a pattern of mechanistically related adverse effects is observed across two or more categories in a consistent manner, this can establish biological plausibility and warrant heightened concern for potential harmful effects in humans.[521]

CONCLUDING SCIENTIFIC ISSUES IN THE TORT LAW

Several major points emerge from this and the chapter 3 discussion. Courts can learn much from *Milward v. Acuity Specialty Products* and from the reasoning of scientific committees. (1) Myriad lines of evidence can be scientifically relevant to judgments about toxicity, not simply statistically significant human data. (2) "There is no hierarchy of evidence," and courts should not impose hierarchies. (3) Scientists use inferences to the best explanation to structure their reasoning, integrate different lines of evidence (by assessing the quality of the relevant and available data), and determine whether and how the different lines of evidence contribute to the conclusion.[522] They should be permitted to do so in legal testimony, following *Milward* and other courts.[523] It is up to judges and juries how well scientists apply such reasoning in a particular case. (4) Animal studies alone (and certainly with other kinds of data) can be especially powerful. (5) At the IARC, animal data plus strong mechanistic data can even be sufficient for classifying a substance as a known or probable human carcinogen. (For a slightly more detailed suggestion see the notes and text at notes 425–427).

In reviewing evidence in support of testimony, judges should ask, "Are the scientific studies used by an expert *scientifically relevant* to the argument being offered? And do the lines of evidence integrated by experts converge to a *scientific foundation sufficiently reliable to be presented to a jury*?" Recall that trial judges' tasks are to determine the reliability of testimony, not its correctness, which is the jury's task (chapter 3). Were they to try to determine correctness, they could easily be tempted to demand ideal scientific evidence, thus precluding many more litigants, largely plaintiffs, from court.

Judges do not necessarily face an easy task, but it is a more scientifically appropriate one that will better align the tort law with appropriate science to serve compensatory justice.

If the tort law follows this guidance, it will advance the possibility of redress in the tort law by providing litigants with greater possibilities of justice, and perhaps more authoritative legal determinations about toxic products, reducing some ignorance about toxins, and increasing somewhat the deterrent effects of torts. In turn, these will constitute modest steps toward making the world a somewhat safer place from toxic substances via tort law determinations.

CONCLUSION

How much and what kinds of evidence required for public health protections and for redress in the tort law importantly affect our lives. If agencies permit or are forced by some procedures to accede to demands for idealistic evidence, we will be less well protected than we easily could be. If companies create a fog of science that misleads agencies or, worse, uses falsified science to influence their decisions (chapter 1), we will also be less well protected.

If trial judges demand ideal, too much or "doubt-free" evidence, or mistakenly exclude quite relevant evidence, this could preclude redress in the tort law, leaving some wrongfully injured parties uncompensated for injuries caused by others.

Discussions of scientific studies and how scientists reason about them are hidden from most of us. Although it may not seem like a major public policy issue, yet how the administrators of our legal system choose to use science matters quite significantly for ordinary citizens. Their decisions can directly, if invisibly, affect our lives.

Chapter 5

Conclusion

Jeromy Darling, Ken Wamsley, Carla Bartlett, Sandy Guest, Brian Milward, and Wilber Tennant's cattle all were likely harmed because of how existing public health laws governed the use of science. Science used too late or not at all to determine the risks of C8 before employees were exposed resulted in injuries to Jeromy Darling and Ken Wamsley. The absence of premarket testing of C8 meant that there was no information about its toxicity. This in turn permitted a highly toxic substance to be in drinking water, leading to Carla Bartlett's kidney cancer.

Wilbur Tennant's cattle died because C8 should not have been disposed directly into the ground, which ultimately contaminated the stream from which his cows drank. Disposal into a hazardous materials site would almost certainly have been required if C8's toxicity had been understood.

Sandy Guest had the misfortune to use a commercial hair product whose formaldehyde concentrations likely would not have been permitted had a risk assessment on its toxicity been completed in a timely manner. However, as we have seen, at its quickest risk data and health protections can emerge quite slowly. The culprits are postmarket laws that permit ignorance about many products, force researchers to begin with little or no toxicity data, and then invite intransigent opposition while independent scientists and the EPA strive to overcome substantial ignorance and issue improved health protections.

Brian Milward's fate was perhaps less clearly affected by public health laws, but it arguably might have been. Products he used containing benzene, at the time a known human carcinogen, were likely insufficiently reviewed for their toxicity, and apparently there were no warnings that they contained a potent carcinogen. His experience does have a message for the future: when a company or an industry routinely uses a common set of products that might contain the same or similar toxicants, there are reasons to review how joint exposures to them would affect employees.

While science provides reliable procedures for revealing causal relations between exposures and diseases, if they are not used in a timely manner, the results we have seen in previous chapters can occur. Consequently, the fates of most of the people named herein exemplify one of the themes of this book: an important social choice is *when* in the life of a chemical creation the excellent tools of science should be employed to protect the public's health. The laws for pharmaceuticals and pesticides requiring science to be used to identify toxic products before the public has been exposed have protected us far better than postmarket laws.

The 1976 TSCA and some other postmarket public health laws permitted people to be harmed and treated unjustly. They permitted battery against fellow citizens via invasions of untested compounds, as well as minor to modest injuries that are also injustices. Opportunity-truncating harms triggered in fetuses, young children, and adults were perhaps the greatest injustices and likely resulted in substantial suffering. In extreme instances, diseases might have changed lives forever, if people contracted quite serious neurological (e.g., loss of IQ, ADHD, lack of impulse control), reproductive (e.g., cervical, breast, testicular, or prostate cancer), or immune-system disorders. The harms have not been relegated to a single generation: some people have suffered multigenerational diseases, with possible transgenerational effects suggested by experimental studies.

Some leaders—legislators, judges, scientists, and company officers—made intentional and some made unwitting choices that have led to these outcomes. Members of Congress in the 1970s may have enacted the 1976 Toxic Substances Control Act (TSCA) without fully understanding the consequences of their decisions. Perhaps they did not comprehend how biologically active general chemicals could be. They likely did not know how extremely permeable humans are to most chemical creations. Perhaps they believed that postmarket laws, like nuisance laws, could sufficiently protect the public. Perhaps they thought that companies would be good citizens and test their products for toxicity. Unfortunately, these beliefs were mistaken. To the extent that legislators misapprehended the full consequences of their choices, they chose unwittingly.

However, other agents, acting under postmarket laws, knowingly or intentionally contributed to fellow citizens' harm. Some companies chose not to reveal the toxicity of their products. Some chose to remain in ignorance, leaving their products untested. Often, affected companies urged health agencies to act only if they had the best—even ideal or "doubt-free"—evidence, which prolonged any toxic exposures. Some tried to delay public health protections as long as possible, as has occurred with formaldehyde. Some have had long-term campaigns to tout the safety of products that they know are harmful. Others paid hired-gun scientists to claim that their products are not harmful or simply to try to create a scientific record that misleads the literature. Some experts skated on the edge of their disciplines or crossed their boundaries simply to have a good living. Some outright lied about the product in question or about what they knew or did not know. By choosing intentionally, these actors cannot avoid responsibility for their choices.

With the Lautenberg Act Congress has finally and importantly chosen to employ science at the time new chemicals are created (or their uses expanded) from 2016 into the future. As a result adverse effects will more likely be detected before they enter commerce and people are potentially put at risk. Years ago Congress made these decisions for pharmaceuticals and pesticides. Pharmaceuticals are created to be biologically active in the human body, and we voluntarily consume them in prescribed amounts via pills, gases, injections, or intravenous lines. Pesticides are biologically active and disrupt the functioning of insects, fungi, and rodents, inter alia. While they are not designed to enter humans' bodies, and we do not invite them in as with prescription drugs, they enter anyway. In 1996 Congress belatedly realized that pesticides could haphazardly invade us through ingestion, inhalation, and absorption through the skin, resulting in cumulative or aggregative exposures that can be biologically active in humans.

An important contribution of the Lautenberg Act is to recognize that although general chemicals are not created to be biologically active in humans or to enter our bodies, they do both. Research on the developmental origins of disease has found that toxic effects of products are heightened during the earliest stages of life. Researchers have found that this occurs from, among other substances, polychlorinated biphenyls, brominated flame retardants, C8, benzene, bisphenol A, phthalates, and various pesticides, along with lead, mercury, and other heavy metals. Moreover, whatever their origins and however they are incorporated into products, these substances too often migrate from cosmetics, plastics, hydraulic fluids, upholstery, frying pans, or factories into the environment and then into human bodies, exemplifying Rachel Carson's concern (see chapter 1). This was Carla Bartlett's fate. Some products have caused minor to extremely serious harms, including premature death, but the full range of adverse effects will likely remain obscure.

The unexpected biological activity of general chemicals, extreme human permeability, and susceptibility to them that might have been a surprise during the heyday of environmental health legislation we now know is not correct.

However, premarket toxicity testing of general chemicals is far from a cure-all. The legacy of products in commerce that were governed by the 1976 TSCA will remain for decades. The EPA and other public health agencies will be required to identify their toxicity about which little may be known. While the Lautenberg Act specifies deadlines and enforceable actions in reviewing such compounds, the agency faces a daunting, massive, and overwhelming task. In carrying it out public health officials should conduct reviews with care, but modulate any unwise demands for near ideal science before the public can be better protected. They could seek alternative approaches that might expedite assessments, identify toxicants earlier, and reveal subpopulations at risk (this last is required by the Lautenberg act).

Thus, I have argued for a second major theme: *how much* and *what kinds of* scientific evidence are required in these contexts are also important social decisions. They can exacerbate or somewhat ameliorate the injustices under postmarket laws. Administrators of the public health agencies should not be lobbied into adopting scientific approaches resembling Arthur Furst's idealized suggestions or industry's "doubt-free" science. Both would likely harm or kill more citizens than would the alternative choices that administrators could make. Administrative procedures could be helpfully modified to permit health agencies to assimilate evidence more quickly and to better protect the public's health.

Demands for idealized science and other quite stringent evidentiary requirements have become strategic and tactical weapons, used by those who wish to keep their products in the market longer or to retain the inertia of the manufacturing processes or profits. Some followed more dishonorable strategies.

While the 1976 TSCA has well served the interests of chemical manufacturers and its panoply of experts, it put the rest of us at risk and harmed some citizens. Public health agencies should adopt scientific procedures and any advances in the Lautenberg Act maximally to compensate for 40 years of chemical risks and improve protections.

Protective regulations are not enough—we must also ensure that citizens who are harmed by chemical products can be redressed for their injuries. Currently if citizens suffer injuries traceable to chemical creations, such as lead, methylmercury, asbestos, DES, or benzene (as did Brian Milward), they too often face substantial scientific hurdles in the tort law merely to have the *possibility* of receiving redress for their injuries. Judges should administer expert testimony and its scientific foundations better than some have in the past, in order to give injured parties the possibility of justice.

In the tort law, especially shortly after the *Daubert* decision, judges might well have unknowingly reviewed testimony and its foundations incorrectly, likely due to the influence of litigants in court. They might have required too much or mistaken kinds of evidence for the context: requiring epidemiological studies, and forbidding animal data, mechanistic data, or other studies in support for testimony unless support for the testimony was accompanied by epidemiological data. Some judges perhaps did not act unwittingly; at least one federal judge has suggested to me that particular appellate courts seek to bar plaintiffs from prevailing and any reason will do.

Brian Milward had a close call when Judge O'Toole's *Milward* district court opinion seemed to require epidemiological studies and held that the case was at an end. Mr. Milward's possibility of redress was preserved by the thoughtful and sensitive decision from the First Circuit Court of Appeals, which much better understood the law, science, and scientific reasoning.

Judges can no longer claim to be poorly informed about science and scientific reasoning in testimony for which they have responsibilities. There are some good legal decisions revealing greater scientific sophistication exhibited by some judicial colleagues. The First Circuit in *Milward* and several other courts point the way. Judges can also learn a great deal by understanding how distinguished research institutions such as the International Agency for Research on Cancer and the US National Toxicology Program assess and reason about substances that cause adverse effects in humans. They should recognize the much wider and more varied patterns of scientific evidence that reveal toxic harm to humans.

Judges also have choices that will make a difference to the lives of citizens—even within the boundaries of the *Daubert* trilogy of cases. Will they demand ideal scientific evidence, science without doubt, or require human epidemiological studies with stringent restrictions? Will they recognize and permit experts to reason about scientific evidence as they do in their own work? Will they learn from the First Circuit's *Milward* decision and recognize numerous patterns of evidence that can reveal causation?

Administrators and judges have choices that can better protect the citizens within public health institutions and within the tort law. I have tried to indicate critical decisions for employing science under the law in these two venues to clarify some major options and their consequences. What will they choose? Will they assist in making the world safer from toxic chemical creations?

NOTES

Preface

1. Phi Beta Kappa Society, "Romanell–Phi Beta Kappa Professorship," available at
   https://www.pbk.org/imis15/PBK_Member/PROGRAMS/AWARDS___
   FELLOWSHIPS/Romanell_Professorship/PBK_Member/Programs/
   Awards___Fellowships/Romanell_Professorship.aspx?hkey=2a4f48c1-
   d7e9-4dc6-99f0-0818fd1d2473.
2. Frank R. Lautenberg Chemical Safety for the 21st Century Act, Public Law
   No: 114-182, signed into law, June 22, 2016.

Introduction

1. Sharon Lerner, "The Teflon Toxin: The Case against DuPont," *The Intercept*,
   August 17, 2015, available at https://theintercept.com/2015/08/17/teflon-
   toxin-case-against-dupont/.
2. Sharon Lerner, "The Teflon Toxin: DuPont and the Chemistry of Deception,"
   The Intercept, August 11, 2015, available at https://theintercept.com/2015/08/
   11/dupont-chemistry-deception/.
3. Ibid.
4. Ibid.
5. Ibid.
6. Ibid.

7. Kyle Steenland et al., "Ulcerative Colitis and Perfluorooctanoic Acid (PFOA) in a Highly Exposed Population of Community Residents and Workers in the Mid-Ohio Valley," *Environmental Health Perspectives* 121.8 (2013): 900–5, available at http://dx.doi.org/10.1289/ehp.1206449.

8. Lerner, "The Teflon Toxin: The Case against DuPont."

9. Ibid.

10. Denis Balibouse, "Teflon on Trial: Ohio Woman Wins $1.6mn Lawsuit Alleging DuPont Chemical Led to Cancer," *Reuters*, October 8, 2015, available at https://www.rt.com/usa/318032-dupont-chemical-cancer-lawsuit/.

11. Lerner, "The Teflon Toxin: The Case against DuPont."

12. Ibid.

13. Vaughn Barry et al., "Perfluorooctanoic Acid (PFOA) Exposures and Incident Cancers among Adults Living near a Chemical Plant," *Environmental Health Perspectives* 121.11–12 (2013): 1313–8.

14. Kyle Steenland et al., "Ulcerative Colitis and Perfluorooctanoic Acid (PFOA)," 900–5.

15. Lerner, "The Teflon Toxin: The Case against DuPont."

16. Kellyn S. Betts, "Perfluoroalkyl Acids: What Is the Evidence Telling Us?," *Environmental Health Perspectives* 115.5 (2007): A250–6. doi:10.1289/ehp.115-a250. PMC 1867999

17. Erich Lipton and Rachel Abrams, "The Uphill Battle to Better Regulate Formaldehyde," *New York Times*, May 3, 2015, available at http://nyti.ms/1E83hxM.

18. US Consumer Product Safety Commission, "An Update on Formaldehyde," Publication 725, 2013 Revision 012013, 3–5.

19. Lipton and Abrams, "The Uphill Battle to Better Regulate Formaldehyde."

20. CBS, *60 Minutes*, "Lumber Liquidators linked to Health and Safety Violations," available at http://www.cbsnews.com/news/lumber-liquidators-linked-to-health-and-safety-violations/.

21. Jim Morris, "She Loved Making People Feel Great: Sandy Guest, 55, Hairdresser," Center for Public Integrity, June 29, 2015, available at https://www.publicintegrity.org/2015/06/29/17533/she-loved-making-people-feel-great.

22. National Research Council (NRC), Committee to Review the Formaldehyde Assessment in the National Toxicology Program Report on Carcinogens, *Review of Formaldehyde Assessment in the National Toxicology Program 12th Report on Carcinogens*" (Washington, DC: National Academies Press, 2014), 5–6. See also the International Agency for Research on Cancer (IARC), "Formaldehyde," in *Special Issue: Chemical Agents and Related Occupations, IARC Monographs on the Evaluation of Carcinogenic Risks to Humans* 100F (2012), available at http://monographs.iarc.fr/ENG/Monographs/vol100F/mono100F-430.pdf.

23. NRC, "Review of Formaldehyde Assessment," 7.

24. This is difficult to estimate because an initial analysis was conducted but then discontinued. Following that, new studies had to be taken into account, so the risk assessment was restarted.

25. *60 Minutes*, "Lumber Liquidators Linked to Health and Safety Violations."

26. David Heath, "Meet the 'Rented White Coats' Who Defend Toxic Chemicals," Center for Public Integrity, February 8, 2016, available at https://www.publicintegrity.org/2016/02/08/19223/meet-rented-white-coats-who-defend-toxic-chemicals.

27. Andrew Pollack, "Weed Killer, Long Cleared, Is Doubted," *New York Times*, March 27, 2015, available at http://nyti.ms/1IF01i0; "France Bans Sale of Monsanto Herbicide Roundup in Nurseries, Frankfurt (AFP), June 15, 2015, available at http://www.afp.com/en/news/france-bans-sale-monsanto-herbicide-roundup-nurseries; Zoe Schlanger, "France Bans Sales of Monsanto's Roundup in Garden Centers Three Months after U.N. Calls It a 'Probable Carcinogen,'" *Newsweek*, June 15, 2015, available at http://www.newsweek.com/france-bans-sale-monsantos-roundup-garden-centers-after-un-names-it-probable-343311.

28. Reference available at http://dailynewsdig.com/top-10-slowest-animals-in-the-world/.

29. Lerner, "The Teflon Toxin: The Case against DuPont."

30. Occupational Safety and Health Administration, "OSHA Fact Sheet: Formaldehyde," available at https://www.osha.gov/OshDoc/data_General_Facts/formaldehyde-factsheet.pdf.

31. US Environmental Protection Agency, "Laws and Regulations: Formaldehyde," available at https://www.epa.gov/formaldehyde/laws-and-regulations.

32. Office of the Attorney General, Kamela D. Harris, "Attorney General Kamal D. Harris Announces Settlement Requiring Honest Advertising over Brazilian Blowout Products," January 30, 2012. Sora Song, "Brazilian Blowout Maker Agrees to Warn Consumers about Formaldehyde," *Time*, January 31, 2012, available at http://healthland.time.com/2012/01/31/brazilian-blowout-maker-agrees-to-warn-consumers-about-formaldehyde/.

33. *Milward v. Acuity Specialty Products Group, Inc.*, 664 F.Supp.2d 137 (D.Mass.2009).

34. *Milward v. Acuity Specialty Products Group, Inc.*, 639 F.3d 11 (First Circuit, 2011).

35. John Rawls, *A Theory of Justice*, rev. ed. (Cambridge, MA: Belknap Press of Harvard University Press, 1999), 3.

36. Rawls, *A Theory of Justice*, rev. ed., 3.

37. Frank R. Lautenberg Chemical Safety for the 21st Century Act, Public Law No: 114-182, signed into law, June 22, 2016.

Chapter 1

38. Rachel Carson, *Silent Spring* (New York: Houghton Mifflin, 1962).
39. Eliza Griswold, "How 'Silent Spring' Ignited the Environmental Movement," *New York Times Magazine*, September 21, 2012, available at http://nyti.ms/P3yGKz (quoting then senator Ernest Gruening of Alaska).
40. Lerner, "The Teflon Toxin: DuPont and the Chemistry of Deception."
41. US Congress, Office of Technology Assessment (OTA), *Identifying and Regulating Carcinogens* (Washington, DC: Government Printing Office, 1987), 134.
42. Ibid., 219–20.
43. *Industrial Union Department., AFL-CIO v. Hodgson*, 499 F. 2d 467 (1974).
44. Collegium Ramazzini, "The Collegium Ramazzini Releases Official Position on the Global Health Dimensions of Asbestos and Asbestos-Related Diseases," June 24, 2015available at http://www.collegiumramazzini.org.
45. OTA, *Identifying and Regulating Carcinogens*, 199–200; Carl F. Cranor, *Legally Poisoned: How the Law Puts Us at Risk from Toxicants* (Cambridge, MA: Harvard University Press, 2011), 135–6.
46. William H. Rodgers Jr., *Environmental Law*, 2nd ed. (St. Paul., MN: West, 1994), 112.
47. W. Page Keeton, ed., *Prosser and Keeton on the Law of Torts*, 5th ed., (St. Paul, MN: West, 1992), 617–8.
48. Ibid., 619.
49. Rodgers, *Environmental Law*, 113.
50. Keeton, ed., *Prosser and Keeton on the Law of Torts*, 5th ed., 619–20.
51. Ibid., 622–3, 627–8.
52. Philip J. Hilts, *Protecting America's Health: The FDA, Business, and One Hundred Years of Regulation* (New York: Alfred A. Knopf, 2003), 145.
53. James L. Schardein and Orest T. Macina, *Human Developmental Toxicants: Aspects of Toxicology and Chemistry* (Boca Raton, FL: Taylor & Francis, 2007), 13.
54. Ibid., 158.
55. Cranor, *Legally Poisoned*, 14.
56. Ellen K. Silbergeld, Daniele Mandrioli, and Carl F. Cranor, "Regulating Chemicals: Law, Science, and the Unbearable Burdens of Regulation," *Annual Review of Public Health* 36 (2015): 175–91.
57. US Council on Environmental Quality, *Toxic Substances* (Washington, DC: US Government Printing Office, 1971), 21.
58. Ibid., v, 21.
59. Ibid.
60. D. McCubbins et al., "Administrative Procedures as Instruments of Political Control," *Journal of Law Economics, & Organization* 3.2: 243–77, at 268.

61. Silbergeld, Mandrioli, and Cranor, "Regulating Chemicals," 177–8.
62. Linda-Jo Schierow, "The Toxic Substances Control Act (TSCA): A Summary of the Act and Its Major Requirements," Congressional Research Service, February 2, 2010, 1, 2, 4, available at https://www.fas.org/sgp/crs/misc/RL31905.pdf.
63. Linda-Jo Schierow, *The Toxic Substances Control Act (TSCA): Implementation and New Challenges*, CRS Report RL34118 (Washington, DC: Congressional Research Service, 2007), 2.
64. US Environmental Protection Agency, "EPA's New Chemicals Program under TSCA: The Basics," available at http://www.chemalliance.org/topics/?subsec=27&id=689.
65. John S. Applegate, "Synthesizing TSCA and REACH: Practical Principles for Chemical Regulation Reform," *Ecology Law Quarterly* 35.4 (2009): 721–68.
66. Schierow, *The Toxic Substances Control Act (TSCA): Implementation*, 9.
67. Ibid., 4.
68. Ibid., 14.
69. Ibid., 7.
70. Ibid.
71. US Environmental Protection Agency, "Appendix: The Toxic Substances Control Act: History and Implementation," 111, available at http://www.epa.gov/oppt/newchems/pubs/chem-pmn/appendix.pdf.
72. Applegate, "Synthesizing TSCA and REACH," 118.
73. Schierow, "The Toxic Substances Control Act (TSCA)," 9.
74. US Institute of Medicine, *Identifying and Reducing Environmental Health Risks of Chemicals in Our Society: Workshop Summary* (Washington, DC: National Academies Press, 2014), 32.
75. Keeton, ed., *Prosser and Keeton on the Law of Torts*, 5th ed., 619–20.
76. Lerner, "The Teflon Toxin: The Case against DuPont."
77. Ibid.
78. Bryan A. Garner, ed., *Black's Law Dictionary*, 8th ed., (St. Paul, MN: Thomson/West, 2004), 1631.
79. Lerner, "The Teflon Toxin: How DuPont Slipped Past the EPA," *The Intercept*, August 20 2015, available at https://theintercept.com/2015/08/20/teflon-toxin-dupont-slipped-past-epa/.
80. David A. Eastmond, personal communication, 2012; Myron Melman, personal communication, 2012.
81. NRC, *Toxicity Testing: Strategies to Determine Needs and Priorities* (Washington, DC: National Academy Press, 1984), 3.
82. Eula Bingham and John C. Bailar, personal communications, 2004.
83. US Environmental Protection Agency, "High Production Volume (HPV) Challenge Program," available at http://nepis.epa.gov/Exe/ZyNET.exe/7000052X.TXT?ZyActionD=ZyDocument&Client=EPA&Index=1995+

Thru+1999&Docs=&Query=&Time=&EndTime=&SearchMethod=1&To
cRestrict=n&Toc=&TocEntry=&QField=&QFieldYear=&QFieldMonth=&
QFieldDay=&IntQFieldOp=0&ExtQFieldOp=0&XmlQuery=&File=D%3A
%5Czyfiles%5CIndex%20Data%5C95thru99%5CTxt%5C00000019%5C70
00052X.txt&User=ANONYMOUS&Password=anonymous&SortMethod=
h%7C &MaximumDocuments=1&FuzzyDegree=0&ImageQuality=r75g8/
r75g8/x150y150g16/i425&Display=p%7Cf&DefSeekPage=x&SearchBack=
ZyActionL&Back=ZyActionS&BackDesc=Results%20page&MaximumPage
s=1&ZyEntry=1&SeekPage=x&ZyPURL.

84. Richard Denison, *High Hopes, Low Marks: A Final Report Card on the High Production Volume Chemical Challenge* (Washington, DC: Environmental Defense, 2007), 3–5.

85. US General Accounting Office. *Chemical Regulation: Options Exist to Improve EPA's Ability to Assess Health Risks and Manage Its Chemical Review Program*, GAO-05-458 (Washington, DC: US General Accounting Office, 2005), 18.

86. Joseph H. Guth et al., "Require Comprehensive Safety Data for All Chemicals," *New Solution* 17.3 (2007): 233–58. ("The EPA has very rarely imposed involuntary controls or testing requirements on a new chemical submission. In about 10% (3,500) of PMNs submitted between 1979 and September 2002, the EPA raised questions about chemical safety that have led 'to voluntary negotiated actions, including withdrawal of the PMN, or some type of control or testing agreement' " [240–1].)

87. Schierow, *The Toxic Substances Control Act (TSCA): Implementation*, 9. See also US Environmental Protection Agency, "Assessing and Managing Chemicals under TSCA: TSCA Confidential Business Information," available at https://www.epa.gov/assessing-and-managing-chemicals-under-tsca/tsca-confidential-business-information.

88. Applegate, "Synthesizing TSCA and REACH," 104–105, 115.

89. US General Accounting Office, *Report to Congress: Toxic Substances Control Act, Legislative Changes Could Make the Act More Effective*, GAO/RCED-94-108 (Washington, DC: US General Accounting Office, September 1994), 4.

90. Cranor, *Legally Poisoned*, 111–3.

91. Brenda Eskenazi et al., "*In Utero* and Childhood Polybrominated Diphenyl Ether (PBDE) Exposures and Neurodevelopment in the CHAMACOS Study," *Environmental Health Perspectives* 121.2 (2013): 257–62, available at http://ehp.niehs.nih.gov/wp-content/uploads/2012/11/ehp1205597.pdf.

92. Steven G. Gilbert, "Polybrominated Diphenyl Ethers (PBDEs)," Toxipedia: Connecting Science and People, 2014, available at http://www.toxipedia.org/pages/viewpage.action?pageId=296.

93. Richard Denison (Environmental Defense Fund), email, January 11, 2014.

94. Jiaqi Lan et al., "Toxicity Assessment of 4-Methyl-1-Cyclohexanemethanol and Its Metabolites in Response to a Recent Chemical Spill in West Virginia, USA," *Environmental Science & Technology* 49.10 (2015): 6284–93.

95. David DiMarini, personal communication, 2012.

96. Mark Schleifstein, "Dispersant Used in BP Spill Might Cause Damage to Human Lungs, Fish, Crab Gills, New Study Says," *Times-Picayune*, April 3, 2015, available at http://www.nola.com/environment/index.ssf/2015/04/dispersant_used_in_bp_spill_mi.html.

97. Frederick F. vom Saal et al., "The Estrogenic Endocrine Disrupting Chemical Bisphenol A (BPA) and Obesity," in *Special Issue: Environment, Epigenetics and Reproduction, Molecular and Cellular Endocrinology* 354.1–2 (2012): 74–84.

98. Brian Bienkowski, "BPA Exposure Linked to Changes in Stem Cells, Lower Sperm Production," *Environmental Health News*, January 22, 2015, available at http://www.environmentalhealthnews.org/ehs/news/2015/jan/bpa-exposure-linked-to-changes-in-stem-cells-lower-sperm-production; Brian Bienkowski, "BPA Triggers Changes in Rats That May Lead to Breast Cancer," *Environmental Health News*, July 2, 2014, available at http://www.environmentalhealthnews.org/ehs/news/2014/jul/bpa-mammary-glands; Liz Szabo, "Researchers Raise Concerns about BPA and Breast Cancer: Doctors Sound Alarm about Prenatal Health Hazards," *USA Today*, October 8, 2013, available at http://www.usatoday.com/story/news/nation/2013/10/08/bpa-and-breast-cancer/2834461/.

99. Brian Bienkowski, "Childhood Asthma, BPA Exposure Linked in New Study," *Environmental Health News*, March 1, 2013, available at http://www.environmentalhealthnews.org/ehs/news/2013/asthma-and-bpa.

100. Joe M. Braun et al., "Impact of Early-Life Bisphenol A Exposure on Behavior and Executive Function in Children," *Pediatrics* 128.5 (2011): 873–82, available at http://pediatrics.aappublications.org/content/early/2011/10/20/peds.2011-1335.

101. Breast Cancer Fund, "Bisphenol A (BPA)," available at http://www.breastcancerfund.org/clear-science/radiation-chemicals-and-breast-cancer/bisphenol-a.html (citing several others).

102. Michael Skinner, personal communication, September 20, 2014. Kerry Grens, "Effects of BPA Substitutes," in *Special Issue: Cancer's Grip, The Scientist* 30.4 (2016), available at http://www.the-scientist.com//?articles.view/articleNo/45789/title/Effects-of-BPA-Substitutes/.

103. Sharon Lerner, "New Teflon Toxin Causes Cancer in Lab Animals," *The Intercept*, March 3, 2016, available at https://theintercept.com/2016/03/03/new-teflon-toxin-causes-cancer-in-lab-animals/.

104. NRC, *Risk Assessment in the Federal Government: Managing the Process* (Washington, DC: National Academy Press, 1983).

105. Risk assessments are not as elaborate under technology-based laws, which seek only to identify whether or not a substance is a serious hazard and

then authorize the reduction of the hazard to the lowest level a technology can achieve.

106. NRC, *Risk Assessment in the Federal Government*, 19–20 (summarizes the steps).

107. OTA, *Identifying and Regulating Carcinogens*, 126–7.

108. Ibid., 20.

109. Cranor, *Legally Poisoned*, 8.

110. US Government Accountability Office (GAO), *Chemical Assessments: Low Productivity and New Interagency Review Process Limit the Usefulness and Credibility of EPA's Integrated Risk Information System*, GAO-08-440 (Washington, DC: US Government Accountability Office, March 2008), 40.

111. Samuel M. Goldman et al., "Solvent Exposures and Parkinson Disease Risk in Twins," *Annals of Neurology* 71.6 (2012): 776–84.

112. Mohan Manikkam et al., "Dioxin (TCDD) Induces Epigenetic Transgenerational Inheritance of Adult Onset Disease and Sperm Epimutations," *PLoS ONE* 7.9 (2012): e46249.

113. US GAO, *Chemical Assessments*, 41.

114. US GAO, *Chemical Assessments*, 37–9. See also Lipton and Abrams, "The Uphill Battle to Better Regulate Formaldehyde."

115. US GAO, *Chemical Assessments*, 35.

116. US Institute of Medicine, *Identifying and Reducing Environmental Health Risks of Chemicals in Our Society* (Washington, DC: National Academies Press, 2014), 27.

117. US GAO, *Chemical Regulation*, 9; *Corrosion Proof Fittings v. Environmental Protection Agency*, 947 F.2d 1201 (Fifth Circuit, 1991).

118. US GAO, *Chemical Regulation*, 9; US Institute of Medicine, *Identifying and Reducing Environmental Health Risks*, 28.

119. US Environmental Protection Agency, "U.S. Federal Bans on Asbestos," available at https://www.epa.gov/asbestos/us-federal-bans-asbestos.

120. Sharon Lerner, "The Teflon Toxin: How DuPont Slipped Past the EPA," *The Intercept*, August 20, 2015, available at https://theintercept.com/2015/08/20/teflon-toxin-dupont-slipped-past-epa/.

121. US Environmental Protection Agency, "Lifetime Health Advisories and Health Effects Support Documents for Perfluorooctanoic Acid and Perfluorooctane Sulfonate," EPA-HQ-OW-2014-0138; FRL_XXXX-X, May 19, 2016, available at https://www.epa.gov/sites/production/files/2016-05/documents/pfoa_pfos_prepub_508.pdf.

122. US Environmental Protection Agency, "Effluent Guidelines: Toxic and Priority Pollutants under the Clean Water Act," available at https://www.epa.gov/eg/toxic-and-priority-pollutants-under-clean-water-act#priority.

123. Claudia Copeland, "Toxic Pollutants and the Clean Water Act: Current Issues," CRS Report 93-849, September 21, 1993, 10.

124. US Environmental Protection Agency, "Table of Regulated Drinking Water Contaminants," available at https://www.epa.gov/ground-water-and-drinking-water/table-regulated-drinking-water-contaminants#Organic.

125. US Environmental Protection Agency, "Drinking Water Contaminant Candidate List (CCL) and Regulatory Determination," available at https://www.epa.gov/ccl.

126. Ibid.

127. Rena Steinzor, Wendy Wagner, and Matthew Shudtz, "The IRIS Information Roadblock: How Gaps in EPA's Main Toxicological Database Weaken Environmental Protection," Center for Progressive Reform, June 5, 2009, available at http://www.progressivereform.org/articles/cpr_iris_904.pdf.

128. California Environmental Protection Agency, State Water Resources Control Board, "Perchlorate in Drinking Water," available at http://www.water-boards.ca.gov/drinking_water/certlic/drinkingwater/Perchlorate.shtml.

129. Steinzor et al., "The IRIS Information Roadblock," 11.

130. Ibid.

131. Carl F. Cranor, *Toxic Torts: Science, Law, and the Possibility of Justice*, 2nd ed. (New York: Cambridge University Press, 2016), 106–11.

132. Would companies, faced with having their products tested for toxicity and approved by a public health agency *before* they were permitted to enter commerce, insist on the very highest and best standards of science before this occurred? In a premarket-testing setting, would they portray themselves as scientific angels? This seems unlikely because of the burden of proof to establish the science.

133. Brown & Williamson Tobacco Company, "Smoking and Health Proposal" (Brown & Williamson document 680561778–1786, 1969), available at https://industrydocumentslibrary.ucsf.edu/tobacco/docs/#id=jryf0138; also cited in David Michaels, *Doubt Is Their Product: How Industry's Assault on Science Threatens Your Health* (New York: Oxford University Press, 2012), 275.

134. Jennifer Sass and David Rosenberg, *The Delay Game: How the Chemical Industry Ducks Regulation of the Most Toxic Substances* (New York: Natural Resources Defense Council, 2011), available at https://www.nrdc.org/sites/default/files/IrisDelayReport.pdf; Michaels, *Doubt Is Their Product*,60–78. This point is also nicely illustrated in David Michaels and Celeste Monforton, "How Litigation Shapes the Scientific Literature: Asbestos and Disease among Automobile Mechanics," *Journal of Law and Policy* 15.3 (2008): 1137–69.

135. NRC, *Review of the Formaldehyde Assessment in the National Toxicology Program 12th Report on Carcinogens* (Washington, DC: National Academies Press, 2014), 7.

136. Sass and Rosenberg, *The Delay Game*, 17.

137. Heath, "Meet the 'Rented White Coats' Who Defend Toxic Chemicals".

138. Michaels, *Doubt Is Their Product*, 73.
139. Sheldon Krimsky, "Do Financial Conflicts of Interest Bias Research? An Inquiry into the 'Funding Effect' Hypothesis," *Science, Technology & Human Values* 38.4 (2013): 566–87, at 583, available at http://sth.sagepub.com/content/38/4/566.
140. IARC, *Special Issue: Arsenic, Metals, Fibres and Dusts, IARC Monographs on the Evaluation of Carcinogenic Risks to Humans* 100C (2012), available at http://monographs.iarc.fr/ENG/Monographs/vol100C/index.php; Collegium Ramazzini, "Collegium Ramazzini Statement: Asbestos Is Still With Us; Repeat Call for a Universal Ban," available at http://www.collegium-ramazzini.org/download/15_FifteenthCRStatement(2010).pdf.
141. Jim Morris, "Ford Spent $40 Million to Reshape Asbestos Science," Center for Public Integrity, February 16, 2016, available at http://www.publicintegrity.org/2016/02/16/19297/ford-spent-40-million-reshape-asbestos-science.
142. Ibid.
143. Ibid.
144. Ford Motor Company, Occupational Health and Safety Department, "Industrial Hygiene," February 22, 1995 (with an earlier date of October 14, 1986).
145. Morris, "Ford Spent $40 Million to Reshape Asbestos Science."
146. Jim Morris, "About 'Science for Sale': The Danger of Tainted Science," Center for Public Integrity, February 18, 2016, available at http://www.publicintegrity.org/2016/02/08/19291/about-science-sale. (Articles that are part of the series can be found at this site.)
147. Michaels, *Doubt Is Their Product*, 97–109, especially 100–9.
148. Ibid.
149. Ibid., 146.
150. Ibid., 147.
151. Ibid., 147.
152. Alex Berenson, "First Vioxx Suit: Entryway into a Legal Labyrinth?," *New York Times*, July 11, 2005, available at http://query.nytimes.com/gst/fullpage.html?res=9407E7D81730F932A25754C0A9639C8B63.
153. Michaels, *Doubt Is Their Product*, 147.
154. Ibid., 148.
155. Lerner, "The Teflon Toxin: DuPont and the Chemistry of Deception."
156. Sam Roe and Patricia Callahan, "Distortion of Science Helped Industry Promote Flame Retardants, Downplay the Health Risks," *Chicago Sun Times*, May 9, 2012.
157. Kristen Lombardi, "Benzene and Worker Cancers: An American Tragedy," Center for Public Integrity, December 4, 2014, available at http://www.publicintegrity.org/2014/12/04/16320/benzene-and-worker-cancers-american-tragedy. Lombardy in her article cites this information from the

American Petroleum Institute, Benzene Health Research Consortium, Shanghai Studies, Internal Documents (revealed during discovery in a tort case, 2003).

158. Heath, "Meet the 'Rented White Coats' Who Defend Toxic Chemicals."

159. *Blum v. Merrell Dow Pharmaceuticals*, 33 Phila. Co. Rptr. 193–258, 247 (1996).

160. Natasha Singer and Duff Wilson, "Medical Editors Push for Ghostwriting Crackdown," *New York Times*, September 17, 2009, available at http://www.nytimes.com/2009/09/18/business/18ghost.htm.

161. *United States of America v. Philip Morris USA, Inc., et al.*, 449 F.Supp.2d 1 (D.D.C. 2006), at 1–2.

162. Michaels and Monforton, "How Litigation Shapes the Scientific Literature."

163. US Council on Environmental Quality, *Toxic Substances*, v.

164. Morris, "Ford Spent $40 Million to Reshape Asbestos Science"; Lerner, "The Teflon Toxin: DuPont and the Chemistry of Deception."

Chapter 2

165. Mayo Clinic Staff, "Diseases and Conditions: Infectious Diseases," available at http://www.mayoclinic.org/diseases-conditions/infectious-diseases/basics/definition/con-20033534.

166. Bruce P. Lanphear, "Origins and Evolution of Children's Environmental Health," in *Special Issue: Essays on the Future of Environmental Health Research: A Tribute to Kenneth Olden, Environmental Health Perspectives* 113 (August 2005): 2.

167. Ibid.

168. Lanphear, ibid.; Philippe Grandjean et al., "The Faroes Statement: Human Health Effects of Developmental Exposure to Chemicals in Our Environment," *Basic & Clinical Pharmacology & Toxicology* 102.2 (2008): 73–5, at 74.

169. Philippe Grandjean et al., "The Faroes Statement," 74

170. Ibid.

171. Cranor, *Legally Poisoned*, 123.

172. I. Caroline McMillen and Jeffrey S. Robinson, "Developmental Origins of the Metabolic Syndrome: Prediction, Plasticity, and Programming," *Physiological Review* 85.2 (2005): 571–633, at 609.

173. Ibid.

174. Johan G. Eriksson et al., "Catch-Up Growth in Childhood and Death from Coronary Heart Disease: Longitudinal Study," *British Medical Journal* 318.7181 (1999): 427–31.

175. McMillen and Robinson, "Developmental Origins of the Metabolic Syndrome," 609.

176. Jerrold J. Heindel, "Animal Models for Probing the Developmental Basis of Disease and Dysfunction Paradigm," *Basic & Clinical Pharmacology & Toxicology* 102.2 (2008): 76–81, at 78.

177. Ibid.

178. Ibid.

179. Mohan Manikkam et al., "Transgenerational Actions of Environmental Compounds on Reproductive Disease and Identification of Epigenetic Biomarkers of Ancestral Exposures," *PLoS ONE* 7.2 (2012): e31901.

180. US Environmental Protection Agency, Office of Pesticide Programs, *General Principles for Performing Aggregate Exposure and Risk Assessments*, November 28, 2001, available at https://www.epa.gov/sites/production/files/2015-07/documents/aggregate.pdf (emphasis in original).

181. Ibid.

182. US Institute of Medicine, *Identifying and Reducing Environmental Health Risks*, 10.

183. Robert W. Gale et al., "Semivolatile Organic Compounds in Residential Air along the Arizona-Mexico Border," *Environmental Science & Technology* 43.9 (2009): 3054–3060.

184. Donald T. Wigle and Bruce P. Lanphear, "Human Health Risks from Low-Level Environmental Exposures: No Apparent Safety Thresholds," *PLoS Medicine* 2.12 (2005): e350; Richard L. Canfield et al., "Low-Level Lead Exposure, Executive Functioning, and Learning in Early Childhood," *Child Neuropsychology* 9.1 (2003): 35–53; Ana Navas-Acien et al., "Lead Exposure and Cardiovascular Disease—a Systematic Review," *Environmental Health Perspectives* 115.3 (2007): 472–82.

185. J. William Langston and Phillip A. Ballard Jr., "Parkinson's Disease in a Chemist Working with 1-Methyl-4-Phenyl-1,2,5,6-Tetrahydropyridine," *New England Journal of Medicine* 309.5 (1983): 310.

186. Tracey J. Woodruff et al., "Environmental Chemicals in Pregnant Women in the United States: NHANES 2003–2004," *Environmental Health Perspectives* 119.6 (2011): 878–85; American College of Obstetricians and Gynecologists Committee on Health Care for Underserved Women, American Society for Reproductive Medicine Practice Committee, with the assistance of the University of California at San Francisco (UCSF) Program on Reproductive Health and the Environment, "Committee Opinion: Exposure to Toxic Environmental Agents," Committee Opinion 575, October 2013.

187. Woodruff et al., "Environmental Chemicals in Pregnant Women in the United States," 878–85.

188. Ibid.

189. American College of Obstetricians and Gynecologists Committee on Health Care for Underserved Women, "Committee Opinion: Exposure to Toxic Environmental Agents."

190. James L. Schardein, *Chemically Induced Birth Defects*, 3rd ed., rev. and expanded (New York: Marcel Dekker, 2000), 5.

191. Peter Wick et al., "Barrier Capacity of Human Placenta for Nanosized Materials," *Environmental Health Perspectives* 118.3 (2010): 432–6.

192. Roy R. Gerona et al. "Bisphenol-A (BPA), BPA Glucuronide, and BPA Sulfate in Midgestation Umbilical Cord Serum in a Northern and Central California Population," *Environmental Science & Technology* 47.21 (2013): 12477–85, available at http://dx.doi.org/10.1021/es402764d; Muna S. Nahar et al., "Fetal Liver Bisphenol A Concentrations and Biotransformation Gene Expression Reveal Variable Exposure and Altered Capacity for Metabolism in Humans," in *Special Issue: National Institute of Environmental Health Sciences Outstanding New Environmental Scientist Program, Journal of Biochemical and Molecular Toxicology* 27.2 (2013): 116–23.

193. Peter Fimrite, "Study: Chemicals, Pollutants Found in Newborns," *SFGate*, December 3, 2009, available at http://www.sfgate.com/health/article/Study-Chemicals-pollutants-found-in-newborns-3207709.php. See also Environmental Working Group, "Pollution in People: Cord Blood Contaminants in Minority Newborns," 2009, available at http://static.ewg.org/reports/2009/minority_cord_blood/2009-Minority-Cord-Blood-Report.pdf?_ga=1.260191565.19537483.1425936452.

194. Mark D. Miller et al., "Differences between Children and Adults: Implications for Risk Assessment at California EPA," *International Journal of Toxicology* 21.5 (2002): 403–18, at 412.

195. Shun'ichi Honda et al., "Recent Advances in Evaluation of Health Effects on Mercury with Special Reference to Methylmercury—a Minireview," *Environmental Health and Preventive Medicine* 11.4 (2006): 171–6, at 176; Birger G. J. Heinzow, "Endocrine Disruptors in Human Breast Milk and the Health-Related Issues of Breastfeeding," in *Endocrine-Disrupting Chemicals in Food*, ed. Ian Shaw (Cambridge, UK: Woodhead, 2009), 322–55, at 324–5 and 322–47.

196. David Bellinger and Herbert L. Needleman, "The Neurotoxicity of Prenatal Exposure to Lead: Kinetics, Mechanisms and Expressions," in *Prenatal Exposure to Toxicants*, ed. Herbert L. Needleman and David Bellinger (Baltimore: Johns Hopkins University Press 1994), 89–111, at 92.

197. Heinzow, "Endocrine Disruptors in Human Breast Milk," 322–55, at 324–5 and 322–47; Philippe Grandjean et al., "Elimination Half-Lives of Polychlorinated Biphenyl Congeners in Children," *Environmental Science & Technology* 42.18 (2008): 6991–6, at 6991.

198. Philippe Grandjean et al., "The Faroes Statement," 73.

199. Ronald D. Hood, "Principles of Developmental Toxicology Revisited," in *Developmental and Reproductive Toxicology: A Practical Approach*, 2nd ed., ed. Ronald D. Hood (Boca Raton, FL: Taylor & Francis, 2006): 3–17, at 7.

200. Cranor, *Legally Poisoned*, 98–9; Rodney R. Dietert and Michael S. Piepenbrink, "Perinatal Immunotoxicity: Why Adult Exposure Assessment Fails to Predict Risk," *Environmental Health Perspectives* 114.4 (2006): 477–83.

201. Philippe Grandjean and Philip J. Landrigan, "Developmental Neurotoxicity of Industrial Chemicals," *The Lancet* 368.9553 (2006): 2167–78.

202. Rodney R. Dietert and Judith T. Zelikoff, "Identifying Patterns of Immune-Related Disease: Use in Disease Prevention and Management," *World Journal of Pediatrics* 6.2 (2010): 111–8.

203. Frederica P. Perera et al., "Molecular Epidemiologic Research on the Effects of Environmental Pollutants on the Fetus," *Environmental Health Perspectives* 107.S3 (1999): 451–60.

204. Maryse F. Bouchard et al., "Prenatal Exposure to Organophosphate Pesticides and IQ in 7-Year-Old Children," *Environmental Health Perspectives* 119.8 (2011): 1189–95.

205. J. Julvez et al., "Prenatal Methylmercury Exposure and Genetic Predisposition to Cognitive Deficit at Age 8 Years," *Epidemiology* 24.5 (2013): 643–50.

206. US Department of Health and Human Services, Centers for Disease Control and Prevention, "Polychlorinated Dibenzo-p-Dioxins, Polychlorinated Dibenzofurans, and Coplanar and Mono-ortho-substituted Polychlorinated Biphenols," in *Third National Report on Human Exposure to Environmental Chemicals* (Atlanta: US Department of Health and Human Services, Centers for Disease Control and Prevention, 2005), 135, available at http://www.jhsph.edu/research/centers-and-institutes/center-for-excellence-in-environmental-health-tracking/Third_Report.pdf.

207. Tracey J. Woodruff et al., "Meeting Report: Moving Upstream-Evaluating Adverse Upstream End Points for Improved Risk Assessment and Decision-Making," *Environmental Health Perspectives* 116.11 (2008): 1568–75.

208. Ibid.

209. Hilts, *Protecting America's Health*, 144–165; Schardein and Macina, *Human Developmental Toxicants*, 131.

210. Diane Dufour-Rainfray et al., "Fetal Exposure to Teratogens: Evidence of Genes Involved in Autism," *Neuroscience & Biobehavioral Reviews* 35.5 (2011): 1254–65.

211. Shanna H. Swan et al., "Decrease in Anogenital Distance among Male Infants with Prenatal Phthalate Exposure," *Environmental Health Perspectives* 113.8 (2005): 1056–61.

212. Grandjean and Landrigan, "Developmental Neurotoxicity of Industrial Chemicals," 2168.

213. Ibid.

214. Honda et al., "Recent Advances in Evaluation of Health Effects on Mercury," 176; Masazumi Harada, "Minamata Disease: Methylmercury Poisoning in

Japan Caused by Environmental Pollution," *Critical Reviews in Toxicology* 25.1 (1995): 1–24, at 3.

215. Cliona M. McHale and Martyn T. Smith, "Prenatal Origin of Chromosomal Translocations in Acute Childhood Leukemia: Implications and Future Directions," *American Journal of Hematology* 75.4 (2004): 254–7; Mel F. Greaves and Joe Wiemels, "Origins of Chromosome Translocations in Childhood Leukaemia," *Nature Reviews Cancer* 3.9 (2003): 639–49.

216. Julie A. Ross et al., "Epidemiology of Childhood Leukemia, with a Focus on Infants," *Epidemiological Reviews* 16.2 (1994): 243–72.

217. DES Action, "DES Timeline," available at http://www.desaction.org/des-timeline/.

218. US National Institutes of Health, National Cancer Institute, "Diethystilbestrol (DES) and Cancer," available at http://www.cancer.gov/cancertopics/causes-prevention/risk/hormones/des-fact-sheet.

219. Ibid.

220. R.C. Pillard et al., "Psychopathology and Social Functioning in Men Prenatally Exposed to Diethylstilbestrol (DES)," *Psychosomatic Medicine* 55.6 (1993): 485–91.

221. Ibid.

222. Barbara A. Cohn et al., "DDT and Breast Cancer in Young Women: New Data on the Significance of Age at Exposure," *Environmental Health Perspectives* 115.10 (October 2007): 1406–14, at 1406.

223. Barbara A. Cohn, et al., "DDT Exposure in Utero and Breast Cancer," *Journal of Endocrinology & Metabolism* 100.8 (2015): 2865–72.

224. Miller et al., "Differences between Children and Adults: Implications for Risk Assessment at California EPA," at 412 (citing NRC, *Health Effects of Exposure to Low Levels of Ionizing Radiation: BEIR V* [Washington, DC: National Academy Press, 1990]).

225. Ibid.

226. G. Kaati et al., "Cardiovascular and Diabetes Mortality Determined by Nutrition during Parents' and Grandparents' Slow Growth Period," *European Journal of Human Genetics* 10.11 (2002): 682–8.

227. Dietert and Piepenbrink, "Perinatal Immunotoxicity," 477–83. See also Miller et al., "Differences between Children and Adults," at 411.

228. Dietert and Zelikoff, "Identifying Patterns of Immune-Related Disease," 111–8.

229. Dietert and Piepenbrink, "Perinatal Immunotoxicity," 480.

230. Dietert and Zelikoff, "Identifying Patterns of Immune-Related Disease," 114.

231. Luz Claudio et al., "Testing Methods for Developmental Neurotoxicity of Environmental Chemicals," *Toxicology and Applied Pharmacology* 164.1 (2000): 1–14, at 6.

232. Diane Dufour-Rainfray et al., "Fetal Exposure to Teratogens," 1256.

233. Canfield et al., "Low-Level Lead Exposure, Executive Functioning, and Learning in Early Childhood," 35–53,; Bellinger and Needleman, "Intellectual Impairment and Blood Lead Levels," 500–2; and Lanphear, "Origins and Evolution of Children's Environmental Health," 28. Also, David A. Eastmond (Environmental Toxicology, University of California, Riverside), personal communication, February 5, 2016.

234. Fred vom Saal, personal communication, 2011.

235. Laura N. Vandenberg et al., "Hormones and Endocrine-Disrupting Chemicals: Low-Dose Effects and Nonmonotonic Dose Responses," *Endocrine Reviews* 33.3 (2012): 378–455.

236. Matthew D. Anway et al., "Endocrine Disruptor Vinclozolin Induced Epigenetic Transgenerational Adult-Onset Disease," *Endocrinology* 147.12 (2006): 5515–23; Manikkam et al., "Transgenerational Actions of Environmental Compounds on Reproductive Disease and Identification of Epigenetic Biomarkers of Ancestral Exposures"; and Manikkam et al., "Dioxin (TCDD) Induces Epigenetic Transgenerational Inheritance of Adult Onset Disease and Sperm Epimutations," 1–15.

237. Eric Nilsson et al., "Environmentally Induced Epigenetic Transgenerational Inheritance of Ovarian Disease," *PLoS ONE* 7.5 (2012): e36129 and Rebecca Tracey et al., "Hydrocarbons (Jet Fuel JP-8) Induce Epigenetic Transgenerational Inheritance of Obesity, Reproductive Disease and Sperm Epimutations," *Reproductive Toxicology* 36 (April 2013): 104–16.

238. Michael K. Skinner et al., "Ancestral Dichlorodiphenyltrichloroethane (DDT) Exposure Promotes Epigenetic Transgenerational Inheritance of Obesity," *BMC Medicine* 11 (2013): 228–50, available at http://www.ncbi.nlm.nih.gov/pmc/articles/PMC3853586/.

239. Ibid.

240. Emily Anthes, "Hey Would-Be Daddies, How You Take Care of Yourself Plays into the Health of Your Future Children," *Miller-McCune*, December 14, 2010, available at http://www.alternet.org/story/149200/hey_would-be_daddies%2C_how_you_take_care_of_yourself_plays_into_the_health_of_your_future_children.

241. Judith Shulevitz, "Why Fathers Really Matter," Sunday Review, *New York Times*, September 8, 2012, available at http://nyti.ms/QavdtZ.

242. As examples, see "The Nuremberg Code" (1947), and World Medical Association, "Declaration of Helsinki: Ethical Principles for Medical Research Involving Human Subjects," both in *Contemporary Issues in Bioethics*, 6th ed., ed. Tom L. Beauchamp and LeRoy Walters (Belmont, CA: Wadsworth, 2003), 354–63.

243. Rawls, *A Theory of Justice*, rev. ed., 53.

244. Ibid.

245. B. Bakke et al., "Uses of and Exposure to Trichloroethylene in U.S. Industry: A Systematic Literature Review," *Journal of Occupational Environmental Hygiene* 4.5 (2007): 375–90; Steven Gilbert, "Trichloroethylene," Toxipedia: Connecting Science and People, 2014, available at http://www.toxipedia. org/display/toxipedia/Trichloroethylene.

246. US Department of Health and Human Services, Centers for Disease Control and Prevention, Agency for Toxic Substances and Disease Registry, Environmental Health and Medicine Education, "Trichloroethylene Toxicity: What Are the Physiological Effects of Trichloroethylene?," November 8, 2007, available at http://www.atsdr.cdc.gov/csem/csem. asp?csem=15&po=10.

247. US Environmental Protection Agency, "Trichloroethylene: Hazard Summary—Created in April 1992; Revised in January 2000,"available at https://www3.epa.gov/airtoxics/hlthef/tri-ethy.html.

248. IARC, "Trichloroethylene," in *Special Issue: Trichloroethylene, Tetrachloroethylene, and Some Other Chlorinated Agents, IARC Monographs on the Evaluation of Carcinogenic Risks to Humans* 106 (2014): 35–218, at 189, available at http://monographs.iarc.fr/ENG/Monographs/vol106/mono106-001.pdf.

249. Goldman et al., "Solvent Exposures and Parkinson Disease Risk in Twins," 776–84.

250. Rawls, *A Theory of Justice*, rev. ed., 63.

251. Norman Daniels, "Health-Care Needs and Distributive Justice," *Philosophy and Public Affairs* 10.2 (1981): 146–79, 167–8.

252. *Mink v. University of Chicago,* 460 F. Supp. 713, 715 (1978).

253. Mary L. Lyndon, "The Toxicity of Low-Dose Chemical Exposures: A Status Report and a Proposal: Review of *Legally Poisoned: How the Law Puts Us at Risk from Toxicants*," *Jurimetrics* 52.4 (2012): 457–500, at 491.

254. *Mink v. Univ. of Chi.,* at 717–8 (citing William Prosser, *Handbook of the Law of Torts*, 4th ed. [St. Paul, MN: West, 1971], at 35; and *Cathemer v. Hunter,* 27 Ariz.App. 780, 558 P.2d 975, 978 [1976]).

255. American Law Institute, *Restatement (Second) of Torts*, §§ 13, 18 (1965).

256. Keeton, ed., *Prosser and Keeton on the Law of Torts*, 5th ed., 39–41.

257. Lyndon, "The Toxicity of Low-Dose Chemical Exposures," 488.

258. *Mink v. Univ. of Chi.,* 460 F. Supp. 713, at 716.

259. Danuta Mendelson, "Historical Evolution and Modern Implications of Concepts of Consent to, and Refusal of, Medical Treatment in the Law of Trespass," *Journal of Legal Medicine* 17.1 (1996): 1–71, at 5.

260. Consent would be difficult or impossible for every "unreasonable" unwanted invasion by an untested substance. However, a plausible surrogate for consent

might require that those who create foreign substances that invade our bodies take reasonable steps to ensure that they are not risky. I considered some of these issues in "Do You Want to Bet Your Children's Health on Postmarket Harm Principles? An Argument for a Trespass or Permission Model for Regulating Toxicants," *Villanova Environmental Law Journal* Vol. 19.2 (2008): 251–314.

261. Lyndon, "The Toxicity of Low-Dose Chemical Exposures," 490.
262. Ibid., 496. See also Ibid., 495.
263. Cranor, *Legally Poisoned*, 183–4.
264. Lyndon, "The Toxicity of Low-Dose Chemical Exposures," 491.
265. Ibid., 497.
266. Rawls, *A Theory of Justice*, rev. ed., 72.
267. Carl F. Cranor, "Risk Assessment, Susceptible Subpopulations, and Environmental Justice," in *The Law of Environmental Justice: Theories and Procedures to Address Disproportionate Risks*, 2nd ed., ed. Michael B. Gerrard and Sheila R. Foster (Chicago: American Bar Association, 2008), 341–94.
268. Max Neiman, *Defending Government: Why Big Government Works* (Upper Saddle River, NJ: Prentice Hall, 2000), 192.
269. Leonardo Trasande and Yinghua Liu, "Reducing the Staggering Costs of Environmental Disease in Children, Estimated at $76.6 Billion in 2008," *Health Affairs* 30.5 (2011): 863–70.
270. Cranor, *Legally Poisoned*, 178–207.
271. Ibid., 194.
272. See, generally, European Community, Registration, Evaluation, Authorisation, and Restriction of Chemicals (REACH), establishing a European Chemicals Agency, December 18, 2006, no. 1907/2006 (United Kingdom) (hereafter, REACH). For a more accessible generic guide, see http://www.reach- serv.com/index.php?option=com_content&task=view &id=121&Itemid=128. Also, for a somewhat more detailed discussion of REACH, see Cranor, *Legally Poisoned*, at 197–99.
273. REACH, Regulation (EC) no. 1907/2006, art. 5.
274. Ibid., art. 1, ¶ 19–21. On number and types of testing and cumulative tests, see art. 1, ¶ 28–9.
275. See REACH, at art. L 396/339, L 396/352-53, L 396/3643-66
276. REACH, O. J. (L 396) 1, 20 (EC),
277. REACH, art. 1, ¶ 28–9.
278. NRC, Committee on Toxicity Testing and Assessment of Environmental Agent, *Toxicity Testing for Assessment of Environmental Agents: Interim Report* (Washington, DC: National Academies Press, 2006), 181.
279. Ibid., 186.
280. Ibid., 186.

Chapter 3

281. *Daubert v. Merrell Dow Pharmaceuticals, Inc.*, 509 U.S. 579 (1993); *General Electric v. Joiner*, 522 U.S. 136 (1997); *Kumho Tire Co., Ltd. v. Carmichael*, 526 U.S. 137 (1999).

282. Cranor, *Toxic Torts*, 2nd ed.

283. Tony Honoré, "The Morality of Tort Law—Questions and Answers," in *Philosophical Foundations of Tort Law*, ed. David G. Owen (Oxford: Clarendon, 1995), 79; Lawrence M. Friedman, *History of American Law*, 2nd ed. (New York: Touchstone, 1985), 470–7.

284. Kim M. Cecil et al., "Decreased Brain Volume in Adults with Childhood Lead Exposure," *PLoS Medicine* 5.5 (2008): pp. 741–50; Ana Navas-Acien et al., "Lead Exposure and Cardiovascular Disease—a Systematic Review," *Environmental Health Perspectives* 115.3 (2007): 472–82.

285. Wigle and Lanphear, "Human Health Risks from Low-Level Environmental Exposures," 1–3; Canfield et al., "Low-Level Lead Exposure and Executive Functioning," 35–53; Bellinger and Needleman, "Intellectual Impairment and Blood Lead Levels," 349; Ellen K. Silbergeld and Virginia M. Weaver, "Exposures to Metals: Are We Protecting the Workers?," *Occupational & Environmental Medicine* 64.3 (2007): 141–2, at 141.

286. David A. Lieb, "Doe Run Settles Lead Liability Cases in Missouri," *Insurance Journal*, September 19, 2013, available at http://www.insurancejournal.com/news/midwest/2013/09/19/305722.htm, last viewed April 4, 2016.

287. Donna Walter, "Missouri Lawyers of the Year Win $358M Toxic Tort Case," *Missouri Lawyer*, January 27, 2012, available at http://molawyersmedia.com/2012/01/27/video-missouri-lawyers-of-the-year/.

288. Clayton P. Gillette and James E. Krier, "Risk, Courts, and Agencies," *University of Pennsylvania Law Review* 138.4 (1990): 1027–1109, at 1046.

289. Ibid., 1045 (emphasis in original).

290. Ibid., 1044 (emphasis in original).

291. Ibid., at 1046.

292. Ibid.

293. IARC, *Special Issue: Some Aromatic Amines, Organic Dyes, and Related Exposures*, IARC Monographs on the Evaluation of Carcinogenic Risks to Humans 99 (2010): 294–5, available at https://monographs.iarc.fr/ENG/Monographs/vol99/mono99.pdf.

294. Ibid.

295. Ibid.

296. Public health agencies have scientific personnel to conduct studies, if need be. They can also interpret others' study results and in general can provide guidance to administrative lawyers about how to make the best scientific case

for protecting the public. Public health scientists would also be part of the decision making about protecting the public.

Tort law firms typically do not have a panoply of in-house experts to address esoteric causal issues. They likely collaborate frequently with a variety of toxicologists, epidemiologists, exposure experts, and industrial hygienists, but this coterie of needed experts is not an organization. Instead they likely seek out experts as needed for particular cases.

297. Michael D. Green et al., "Reference Guide on Epidemiology," in *Reference Manual on Scientific Evidence*, 2nd ed., ed. Federal Judicial Center (Washington, DC: Federal Judicial Center, 2000), at 570.

298. *Hurtado v. Pharma Co.*, 6 Misc.3d 1015(A), 2005 WL 192351 (N.Y. Sup. Ct. 2005), at 6.

299. Kathleen Michon, "Toxic Tort Litigation: Common Defenses," Nolo Law for All, available at http://www.nolo.com/legal-encyclopedia/toxic-tort-litigation-common-defenses-32209.html.

300. Gillette and Krier, "Risk, Courts, and Agencies," 1046.

301. Jonathan Harr, *A Civil Action* (New York: Vintage, 1996).

302. Michael J. Saks, "Do We Really Know Anything about the Behavior of the Tort Litigation System—and Why Not?," *University of Pennsylvania Law Review* 140.4 (1992): 1147–292, at 1189.

303. Gillette and Krier, "Risk, Courts, and Agencies," 1056.

304. Ibid., 1054.

305. Ibid., 1055.

306. Ibid., 1056–7. ("Consider in this respect the handful of cases that so concerns some of the courts' critics. Any one or all of these can readily enough be criticized for subjecting particular public risk producers to unduly harsh treatment. Such expansive liability can drive relatively safe enterprises out of the market, and in this sense the decisions in question are costly.... [However,] by inflating the liability imposed on *any* public risk producer brought to judgment, process bias increases the expected liability that must be anticipated by *all* public risk producers in the market, so long as public risk claims enter the liability system on an essentially random basis. On this view, the social costs resulting from inflated liability in any particular case are simply the premium paid for the service of augmenting expected values that are probably otherwise too low. The enhanced recoveries amplify a signal that is weak at its origin. The premium exacted in the process may be unavoidable, and in any event worthwhile" [at 1057].)

307. Saks, "Do We Really Know Anything about the Behavior of the Tort Litigation System," 1147–289.

308. Ibid., 1183.

309. Ibid., 1184–5.

310. Ibid., 1186. ("[M]alpractice cases ought to be the most difficult ones for the system to handle. If the system can handle medical malpractice with reasonable "accuracy," it probably can handle almost anything." Ibid., 1226.)

311. Ibid., 1189.
312. Ibid., 1189.
313. Ibid., 1185.
314. Ibid., 1226.
315. Ibid., 1286.
316. *Frye v. U.S.* 54 App. D.C. 46 (1923).
317. *Donaldson v. Central Illinois Public Service*, 767 N.E.2d 314 at 325 (2002).
318. *Daubert v. Merrell Dow Pharmaceuticals, Inc.*, 509 U.S. 579 (1993).
319. Michael D. Green, *Bendectin and Birth Defects: The Challenges of Mass Toxic Substances Litigation* (Philadelphia: University of Pennsylvania Press, 1996), 129.
320. *Daubert v. Merrell Dow Pharmaceuticals, Inc.*, 727 F.Supp. 570 (1989), at 573.
321. See Ibid., at 575.
322. *Daubert v. Merrell Dow Pharm., Inc.*, 951 F.2d 1128 (9th Cir. 1991).
323. *Daubert v. Merrell Dow Pharm., Inc.*, 43 F.3d 1311 (9th Cir. 1995).
324. *Daubert v. Merrell Dow Pharm., Inc.*, 509 U.S. 588–9.
325. Ibid.
326. Ibid., 596.
327. *Brock v. Merrell Dow Pharmaceuticals, Inc.*, 874 F.2d 307 (5th Cir. 1989). ("Undoubtedly, the most useful and conclusive type of evidence in a case such as this is epidemiological studies"; at 311.)
328. Advisory Committee on Evidence Rules, "Proposed Amendment: Rule 702" (December 2011), available at http://www.law.cornell.edu/rules/fre/rule 702.
329. Some articles critically assessing the effects of the *Daubert* trilogy on the law include Carl F. Cranor et al., "Judicial Boundary Drawing and the Need for Context-Sensitive Science in Toxic Torts after *Daubert v. Merrell Dow Pharmaceutical*," *Virginia Environmental Law Journal* 16 (1996): 1–77; Margaret A. Berger, "The Supreme Court's Trilogy on the Admissibility of Expert Testimony," in *Reference Manual on Scientific Evidence*, 2nd ed., ed. Federal Judicial Center (Washington, DC: Federal Judicial Center, 2000); Lucinda M. Finley, "Guarding the Gate to the Courthouse: How Trial Judges are Using Their Evidentiary Screening Role to Remake Tort Causation Rules," *DePaul University Law Review* 49.2 (1999): 335–77; Michael H. Graham, "The Expert Witness Predicament: Determining 'Reliable' under the Gatekeeping Test of *Daubert, Kumho*, and Proposed Amended Rule 702 of the Federal Rules of Evidence," *University of Miami Law Review* 54.2 (2000): 317–57; Michael D. Green, "The Road Less Well Traveled (and Seen): Contemporary Lawmaking in Products Liability," *DePaul Law Review* 49.2 (1999): 377–403; Carl F. Cranor and David A. Eastmond, "Scientific Ignorance and Reliable Patterns of Evidence in Toxic Tort Causation: Is There a Need for Liability Reform?," in *Special Issue: Causation in Law and Science, Law and Contemporary Problems* 64.4

(2001), 5–48; and Carl F. Cranor, "A Framework for Assessing Scientific Arguments: Gaps, Relevance and Integrated Evidence," *Journal of Law and Policy*, 15.1 (2007): 7–58.

330. Finley, "Guarding the Gate to the Courthouse."

331. Ibid.

332. *General Electric v. Joiner*, 522 U.S. 136 (1997).

333. *General Electric v. Joiner*, 522 U.S. 142. ("A court of appeals applying "abuse-of-discretion" review . . . may not categorically distinguish between rulings allowing expert testimony and rulings disallowing it.")

334. *General Electric v. Joiner*, 522 U.S. 146–7.

335. Margaret A. Berger, "The Admissibility of Expert Testimony," in *Reference Manual on Scientific Evidence*, 3rd ed., ed. Federal Judicial Center (Washington, DC: National Academies Press, 2011), 19.

336. Sheldon Krimsky, "The Weight of Scientific Evidence in Policy and Law," *American Journal of Public Health* 95.S1 (2005): S129–36, at S129.

337. James D. Watson and Francis H. C. Crick, "Molecular Structure of Nucleic Acids: A Structure for Deoxyribose Nucleic Acid," *Nature* 171.4356 (1953): 737–8.

338. Susan Haack, "An Epistemologist in the Bramble-Bush: At the Supreme Court with Mr. Joiner," *Journal of Health Politics, Policy and Law* 26 (2001): 217–237.

339. Cranor, *Toxic Torts*, 2nd ed., 338–43.

340. *Kumho Tire Co., Ltd. v. Carmichael*, 526 U.S. 137 (1999).

341. Ibid., at 152.

342. Ibid., at 154 (citing *Daubert* at 596).

343. Cranor, *Toxic Torts*, 2nd ed., 219–50.

344. Ibid., 129–48, 295–304.

345. Greg Winter, "Jury Awards Soar as Lawsuits Decline on Defective Goods," *New York Times*, January 30, 2001, available at http://www.nytimes.com/2001/01/30/business/30JURY.html?pagewanted=all.

346. Ibid.

347. Ibid.

348. Ibid.

349. Bruce Kaufman, "Daubert Exclusions 'Haunt' Experts, but Need Not Be Career Ending Blows," *Bloomberg Occupational & Health Reporter* 46.14 (2016): 343–6.

350. Andrew W. Jurs and Scott DeVito, "The Stricter Standard: An Empirical Assessment of *Daubert*'s Effect on Civil Defendants," *Catholic University Law Review* 62.3 (2013): 675–731.

351. Andrew W. Jurs and Scott DeVito, "Et Tu, Plaintiffs? An Empirical Analysis of *Daubert*'s Effect on Plaintiffs, and Why Gatekeeping Standards Matter (a Lot)," *Arkansas Law Review* 66.4 (2013): 975–1006.

352. *Milward v. Acuity Specialty Products*, 639 F.3d 11 (2011).
353. Carl F. Cranor, *Toxic Torts*, 2nd ed.,128–44, 286–94; Cranor and Eastmond, "Scientific Ignorance and Reliable Patterns of Evidence," 5–48; Cranor, "A Framework for Assessing Scientific Arguments," 7–58; and Carl F. Cranor, "Scientific Inferences in the Laboratory and the Law," in *Special Issue: Scientific Evidence and Public Policy, American Journal of Public Health* 95.S1 (2005): S121–8.
354. Martyn T. Smith, "Declaration of Martyn T. Smith," in *Milward v. Acuity Specialty Products*, March 9, 2009.
355. *Harris v. CSX Transp., Inc.*, 753 S.E.2d 275, 287–9, W.Va., November 13, 2013 (the Supreme Court of West Virginia accepted all the main points of the *Milward* decision); *Loewen v. Wyeth, Inc.* (not reported in F.Supp.2d, 2011) WL 6140889, at 5 (N.D.Ala., 2011); *In re Chantix (Varenicline) Products Liability*, 889 F.Supp.2d 1272, at 1300 (N.D.Ala.,2012); *In re Fosamax (Alendronate Sodium) Products Liability* (not reported in F.Supp.2d, 2013 WL 1558690), at 4 (D.N.J.,2013); and *Johns v. Bayer Corp.*, 2013 WL 1498965, at 21 (S.D. Cal. Apr. 10, 2013).
356. *Milward v. Acuity Specialty Products*, 639 F.3d., at 22–3.
357. Ibid., at 15 (quoting *Ruiz-Troche v. Pepsi Cola of P.R. Bottling Co.*, 161 F.3d 77, 85 [1st Cir. 1998]).
358. Ibid., at 15, 26.
359. Ibid., 15.
360. Ibid.
361. Ibid., at 23.
362. Ibid., at 19.
363. Ibid., at 17.
364. Ibid., at 18–9.
365. Ibid., at 19, (citing *Kumho Tire*).
366. Nathan A. Schachtman, "WOE-fully Inadequate Methodology—an Ipse Dixit by Another Name," available at http://schachtmanlaw.com/woe-ful-inadequate-methodology-an-ipse-dixit-by-another-name/, last viewed 4/4/2016.
367. *Milward v. Acuity Specialty Products*, 639 F.3d at 18 (citing Restatement of Torts, § 28 cmt. c[1]).
368. *Milward v. Acuity Specialty Products, Inc.*, 664 F.Supp. 2d 148.
369. *Milward v. Acuity Specialty Products*, 639 F.3d at 24.
370. *U.S. Steel Corp. v. Milward*, 132 S.Ct. 1002 (2012).
371. Lombardi, "Benzene and Worker Cancers."
372. Saks, "Do We Really Know Anything about the Behavior of the Tort Litigation System," 1218.
373. *Kumho Tire Co., Ltd. v. Carmichael*, 526 U.S. 154.
374. *Kumho Tire Co., Ltd. v. Carmichael*, 526 U.S. 153 (citing *Daubert* at 596).

375. Cranor, *Toxic Torts*, 2nd ed., 286–324; Cranor and Eastmond, "Scientific Ignorance and Reliable Patterns of Evidence," 5–48; Cranor, "A Framework for Assessing Scientific Arguments," 7–58; and Cranor, "Scientific Inferences in the Laboratory and the Law," 121–8.

376. Of course, we do not know what a jury would have decided. However, plaintiffs whose trial ended because a judge mistakenly ruled that scientific testimony was unreliable were denied the *possibility* of justice.

Chapter 4

377. Public health agencies could show variation in how much evidence they demand because they are subject to different laws—some requiring more-demanding scientific showings, others less so. Agencies may also have varying degrees of latitude under "arbitrary and capricious" procedures compared with "substantial evidence" procedures.

378. Cranor, *Legally Poisoned*, 7, 10, 133, 168–77.

379. Charles Nesson, "The Evidence or the Event? On Judicial Proof and the Acceptability of Verdicts," *Harvard Law Review* 98.7 (1985): 1357–92.

380. Arthur Furst, "Yes, but Is It a Human Carcinogen?," *Journal of the American College of Toxicology* 9.1 (1990), 1–18, at 12.

381. I follow Naomi Oreskes's use of this term. While harsh, it reminds us to think about what mistakes we might make. Naomi Oreskes, "Playing Dumb on Climate Change," *New York Times*, January 3, 2015, available at http://nyti. ms/1F0OIm6, http://www.nytimes.com/2015/01/04/opinion/sunday/playing-dumb-on...on=c-column-top-span-region&WT.nav=c-column-top-span-region&_r=0.

382. For some discussion, see Cranor, *Toxic Torts*, 2nd ed., 184–5.

383. Carl F. Cranor, "The Social Benefits of Expedited Risk Assessments," *Risk Analysis* 15.3 (1995): 353–8.

384. Vincent James Cogliano et al., "The Science and Practice of Carcinogen Identification and Evaluation," *Environmental Health Perspectives* 112.13 (2004): 1269–74, especially 1270; Vincent James Cogliano et al., "Preventable Exposures Associated with Human Cancers," *Journal of the National Cancer Institute* 103.24 (2011): 1827–39.

385. Kurt Straif, "Carcinogens in the Workplace: State of the Art and Future Challenges," presentation in New Delhi, India, March 23, 2011.

386. IARC, "Asbestos (Chrysotile, Amosite, Croccidolite, Tremolite, Actinolite, and Anthophyllite)," in *Special Issue: Arsenic, Metals, Fibres and Dusts, IARC Monographs on the Evaluation of Carcinogenic Risks to Humans* 100C (2012): 294, available at http://monographs.iarc.fr/ENG/Monographs/vol100C/index.php.

387. Cogliano et al., "Science and Practice," 1270.

388. James Huff and David P. Rall, "Relevance to Humans of Carcinogenesis Results from Laboratory Animal Toxicology Studies," in *Maxcy-Rosenau-Last Public Health & Preventive Medicine*, 13th ed., ed. John M. Last and Robert B. Wallace (Norwalk, CT: Appleton & Lange, 1992), 433.

389. Cranor, *Legally Poisoned*, 26–8.

390. Canfield et al., Low-Level Lead Exposure and Executive Functioning," 35–53.

391. Elaine M. Faustman and Gilbert S. Omenn, "Risk Assessment," in *Casarett and Doull's Toxicology: The Basic Science of Poisons*, 6th ed., ed. Curtis D. Klaassen (New York: Pergamon, 2001), 83–104, at 86.

392. NRC, *Review of EPA's Integrated Risk Information System (IRIS) Process* (Washington, DC: National Academy Press, 2014), 85.

393. Cranor and Eastmond, "Scientific Ignorance and Reliable Patterns of Evidence," 5–48.

394. IARC, *List of Classifications* (last updated February 22, 2016), available at http://monographs.iarc.fr/ENG/Classification.

395. Cogliano et al., "Preventable Exposures Associated with Human Cancers," 6.

396. Vincent James Cogliano et al., "Use of Mechanistic Data in IARC Evaluations," *Environmental and Molecular Mutagenesis* 49.2 (2008):100–9, at 103.

397. IARC, *List of Classifications*. See also Carl F. Cranor, "*Milward v. Acuity Specialty Products*: Advances in General Causation Testimony in Toxic Tort Litigation," *Wake Forest Journal of Law & Policy* 3.1 (2013): 132.

398. Carbone et al., "Modern Criteria to Establish Human Cancer Etiology," *Cancer Research* 64.15 (2004): 5519.

399. Guidelines for such inferences have been articulated in IARC, "Preamble," section B.3 ("Studies of Cancer in Experimental Animals"), *IARC Monographs on the Evaluation of Carcinogenic Risks to Humans* http://monographs.iarc.fr/ENG/Preamble/CurrentPreamble.pdf., (rev. 2006), available at. See also Cranor, *Toxic Torts*, 2nd ed., 106–11, 338–43.

400. Carbone et al., "Modern Criteria," 5519.

401. David P. Rall et al., "Alternatives to Using Human Experience in Assessing Health Risks," *Annual Review of Public Health* 8 (1987): 355–85, at 356.

402. Huff and Rall, "Relevance to Humans," 434. ("Significant scientific understanding of neural transmission, renal function, and cell replication and development of cancer have come from non-human species, often species far removed phylogenetically from humans.") James Huff, in "Chemicals and Cancer in Humans: First Evidence in Experimental Animals," *Environmental Health Perspectives* 100 (April 1993): 201, 204, makes an even stronger point: the array and multiplicity of carcinogenic processes are virtually common between laboratory rodents and humans.

403. Huff and Rall, "Relevance to Humans," 433.

404. Bernard D. Goldstein, "Toxic Torts: The Devil Is in the Dose," *Journal of Law and Policy* 16.2 (2009): 551–87, at 556–7.

405. US Department of Health and Human Services, Task Force on Health Risk Assessment, *Determining Risks to Health: Federal Policy and Practice* (Dover, MA: Auburn House, 1986), 10–13; US Congress, Office of Technology Assessment (OTA), *Identifying and Regulating Carcinogens* (Washington, DC: US Government Printing Office, 1987); and NRC, *Risk Assessment in the Federal Government: Managing the Process* (Washington, DC: National Academy Press, 1983).

406. Animal studies use high doses to overcome problems of small sample sizes that are typically used to identify toxicants and to keep costs under control. See NRC, *Risk Assessment in the Federal Government*, 24–27; see also OTA, *Identifying and Regulating Carcinogens*, 39, 46.

407. Cogliano et al., "Use of Mechanistic Data in IARC Evaluations," 108 (the National Toxicology Program identified two such substances out of hundreds reviewed: ethyl acrylate and saccharin).

408. IARC, "Preamble," section B.3, *IARC Monographs on the Evaluation of Carcinogenic Risks to Humans* (rev. 2006).

409. Cogliano et al., "Science and Practice," 1270. ("[A]nimal studies generally provide the best means of assessing particular risks to humans," and studies of the mechanism of action in animals and humans can be utilized to address the pertinence of animals studies to human cancer.)

410. NRC, *Science and Judgment in Risk Assessment* (Washington, DC: National Academy Press, 1994), 58–60.

411. Huff and Rall, "Relevance to Humans," 437. ("[C]hemicals that are carcinogenic in laboratory animals are likely to be carcinogenic in human populations and that, if appropriate studies can be performed, there is qualitative predictability. Also, there is evidence that there can be a quantitative relationship between the amount of a chemical that is carcinogenic in laboratory animals and the amount that is carcinogenic in human populations.")

412. California Environmental Protection Agency, Office of Environmental Health Hazard Assessment, "Guidance Criteria for Identifying Chemicals for Listing as 'Known to the State to Cause Cancer,'" available at http://oehha.ca.gov/prop65/policy_procedure/pdf_zip/revcriteria.pdf.

413. Lorenzo Tomatis et al., "Avoided and Avoidable Risks of Cancer," *Carcinogenesis* 18.1 (1997): 97–105, at 97.

414. US Institute of Medicine (IOM) and NRC, Committee on the Framework for Evaluating the Safety of Dietary Supplements, *Dietary Supplements: A Framework for Evaluating Safety* (Washington, DC: National Academy Press, 2005), 157.

415. Companies' denigrating animal studies may have more influence with the general public, but agency scientists know enough to be able to resist the criticisms.

416. For years the known carcinogen arsenic could not be found to produce cancer in animals. As of 2016, the probable human carcinogen and anticancer drug

etoposide does not cause cancer in experimental animals: IARC, "Etoposide," in *Special Issue: Some Antiviral Drugs, and Other Pharmaceutical Agents, IARC Monographs on the Evaluation of Carcinogenic Risks to Humans* 76 (2000): 177–258, at 238, available at http://www.inchem.org/documents/iarc/vol76/etoposide.html.

417. IARC, "Preamble," section B.4, *IARC Monographs on the Evaluation of Carcinogenic Risks to Humans* (rev. 2006).

418. Cogliano et al., "Use of Mechanistic Data in IARC Evaluations," 103.

419. Ibid.

420. Ibid.

421. Ibid.

422. Ibid., 105.

423. Kenneth S. Santone and Garth Powis, "Mechanism of and Tests for Injuries," in *Handbook of Pesticide Toxicology*, Vol. 1, *General Principles*, ed. Wayland J. Hayes Jr. and Edward R. Laws Jr. (San Diego, CA: Academic Press, 1991), 169.

424. NRC, *Review of EPA's Integrated Risk Information System (IRIS) Process*, 85.

425. Carbone et al., "Modern Criteria," 5522. See also IOM and NRC, *Dietary Supplements: A Framework for Evaluating Safety*, 254. ("It is also not appropriate to develop a hierarchical approach to considering the different types of data—human data, animal data, *in vitro* data or information about related substances—for various reasons. In part, such an approach is not feasible because of limitations in the quality of the data and what different types of studies can reveal, but these limitations can be overcome with other types of data.")

426. IOM and NRC, *Review of EPA's Integrated Risk Information System (IRIS) Process*, 86.

427. This recommendation is similar to one I made for the tort law in Cranor, *Toxic Torts*, 2nd ed., 321–2.

428. U.S. EPA, Assessing and Managing Chemicals under TSCA: Highlights of Key Provisions in the Frank R. Lautenberg Chemical Safety for the 21st Century Act. Available at https://www.epa.gov/assessing-and-managing-chemicals-under-tsca/highlights-key-provisions-frank-r-lautenberg-chemical.

429. Ibid.

430. Ibid.

431. Ibid.

432. Rena Steinzor, "One Step Forward and Two Steps Back on Toxic Chemicals," Center for Progressive Reform. Available at http://www.progressivereform.org/CPRBlog.cfm?idBlog=DCC744AA-DE30-519C-874E812BFA8BE657 and at http://www.huffingtonpost.com/rena-steinzor/crossing-the-rubicon-on-t_b_10110578.html.

433. Ibid.

434. Ibid.

435. Richard Dennison, "Historic deal on TSCA reform reached, setting stage for a new law after 40 years of waiting," Environmental Defense Fund, located at blogs.edf.org/health/2016/05/23/historic-deal-on-tsca-reform-reached-setting-stage-for-a-new-law-after-40-years-of-waiting/#more-5276.

436. Steinzor, "One Step Forward and Two Steps Back on Toxic Chemicals."

437. U.S. EPA, "Highlights of Key Provisions in the Frank R. Lautenberg Chemical Safety for the 21st Century Act."

438. Ibid.

439. The author serves on the Science Guidance Panel of California's Biomonitoring Program.

440. Rachel Morello-Frosch et al., "Understanding the Cumulative Impacts of Inequalities in Environmental Health: Implications for Policy," *Health Affairs* 30.5 (2011): 879–87; and Julia Green Brody et al., "Linking Exposure Assessment Science with Policy Objectives for Environmental Justice and Breast Cancer Advocacy: The Northern California Household Exposure Study," *American Journal of Public Health* 99.S3 (2009):S600–9.

441. Cranor, "Risk Assessment, Susceptible Subpopulations, and Environmental Justice," in *The Law of Environmental Justice*, 2nd ed., 341–94.

442. Carl F. Cranor, "Information Generation and Use under Proposition 65: Model Provisions for Other Postmarket Laws?" *Indiana Law Review* 83.2 (2008): 609–27.

443. Cranor, *Legally Poisoned*, 38.

444. Kim Hooper and Thomas A. McDonald, "The PBDEs: An Emerging Environmental Challenge and Another Reason for Breast-Milk Monitoring Programs," *Environmental Health Perspectives* 108.5 (2000): 387–92, at 388.

445. Ker Than, "Organophosphates: A Common but Deadly Pesticide," *National Geographic Daily News*, July 18, 2013, available at http://news.nationalgeographic.com/news/2013/07/130718-organophosphates-pesticides-indian-food-poisoning/.

446. Woodruff et al., "Meeting Report: Moving Upstream-Evaluating Adverse Upstream End Points for Improved Risk Assessment and Decision-Making," 1568–75.

447. Ronald L. Melnick, "Carcinogenicity and Mechanistic Insights on the Behavior of Epoxides and Epoxide-Forming Chemicals," in *Special Issue: Carcinogenesis Bioassays and Protecting Public Health: Commemorating the Lifework of Cesare Maltoni and Colleagues, Annals of the New York Academy of Sciences* 982 (2002): 177–89.

448. Cogliano et al., "Use of Mechanistic Data in IARC Evaluations," 100–9.

449. Ila Cote et al., "The Next Generation of Risk Assessment Multiyear Study— Highlights of Findings, Applications to Risk Assessment and Future Directions," *Environmental Health Perspectives*, April 19, 2016, available at http://dx.doi.org/10.1289/EHP233.

450. Ibid., 5 (prior to printed version).
451. Carl F. Cranor, "What Could Precautionary Science Be? Research for Early Warnings and a Better Future," in *Precaution: Environmental Science, and Preventive Public Policy*, ed. Joel A. Tickner (Washington, DC: Island, 2003), 305–20.
452. Larry D. Claxton et al., "The *Salmonella* Mutagenicity Assay: The Stethoscope of Genetic Toxicology for the 21st Century," *Environmental Health Perspectives* 118.11 (2010): 1515–22.
453. Sara M. Hoover et al., "Improving the Regulation of Carcinogens by Expediting Cancer Potency Estimation," *Risk Analysis* 15.2 (1995): 267–80; Cranor, "The Social Benefits of Expedited Risk Assessment," 353–8.
454. Hoover et al., "Improving the Regulation of Carcinogens by Expediting Cancer Potency Estimation," 269–70.
455. California Environmental Protection Agency, Office of Environmental Health Hazard Assessment, *Expedited Cancer Potency Values and Proposed Regulatory Levels for Certain Proposition 65 Carcinogens* (Sacramento: California Environmental Protection Agency, Office of Environmental Health Hazard Assessment, April 1992), available at http://oehha.ca.gov/prop65/pdf/exp-cancer.pdf.
456. Cranor, "What Could Precautionary Science Be?," 305–20.
457. Cranor, "Information Generation and Use under Proposition 65," 609–27.
458. Cranor, *Legally Poisoned*, 193. ([C]ompanies that create, manufacture, import, and distribute industrial chemicals that invariably invade humans should be legally required to conduct their business in a manner that will reduce risks and avoid battery and trespass to the public: they should fund or conduct appropriate tests specified by public health agencies (in consultation with independent scientists) in order to identify risks to developing children and people in other sensitive life stages before exposures occur. The battery of tests should aim to ensure that there is a reasonable certainty of no harm to people as a result of contact with the substances in question. The test results should be reviewed by independent scientists before companies are licensed to introduce their products into commerce or to continue marketing products already in commerce. Both new and existing industrial compounds should be evaluated.)
459. NRC, Committee on Toxicity Testing and Assessment of Environmental Agents, *Toxicity Testing for Assessment of Environmental Agents*, 12–13. See also NRC, Committee on Toxicity Testing and Assessment of Environmental Agents, et al., *Toxicity Testing in the 21st Century: A Vision and a Strategy* (Washington, DC: National Academies Press, 2007), 19.
460. *Toxicity Testing for Assessment of Environmental Agents*, 187.
461. Ibid., 190.
462. Cranor, "Do You Want to Bet Your Children's Health on Post-market Harm Principles?," 251–314. (Appropriate required testing could serve as

something of a surrogate for consent, endorsed by the legal system through congressional enactment.)

463. U.S. EPA, "Highlights of Key Provisions in the Frank R. Lautenberg Chemical Safety for the 21st Century Act."

464. Sidney A. Shapiro, "Book Review: *Legally Poisoned*," *American Journal of Industrial Medicine* 55.2 (2012): 187–188, especially 188.

465. Frank Ackerman, "The Unbearable Lightness of Regulatory Costs," *Fordham Urban Law Journal* 33.4 (2006): 1071–1096, at 1077.

466. Trasande and Liu, "Reducing the Staggering Costs of Environmental Disease in Children, Estimated at $76.6 Billion in 2008," 863–70.

467. Ackerman, "The Unbearable Lightness of Regulatory Costs," 1076–7.

468. Cranor, *Legally Poisoned*, 243.

469. Ackerman, "The Unbearable Lightness of Regulatory Costs," 1076–7.

470. *Kumho Tire Co. v. Carmichael*, 526 U.S. 137 (1999) (citing *Daubert v. Merrell Dow Pharm., Inc.*, 509 U.S. 579 [1993]).

471. Cranor, *Toxic Torts*, 2nd ed., 216–53.

472. Cranor, *Toxic Torts*, 2nd ed., 129–54; Cranor, "A Framework for Assessing Scientific Arguments," 7–58.

473. *Wade-Greaux v. Whitehall Lab., Inc.*, 874 F. Supp. 1441, at 1448 (1994).

474. *Wade-Greaux v. Whitehall Lab., Inc.*, 874 F. Supp. 1441, at 1448 (1994).

475. Ibid.

476. *Wade-Greaux v. Whitehall Lab., Inc.*, 874 F. Supp. at 1441 (D.V.I.), *aff'd*, 46 F.3d 1120 (3d Cir. 1994).

477. *Wade-Greaux v. Whitehall Lab., Inc.*, 874 F. Supp. at 1450.

478. Because this case followed shortly after *Daubert*, this judge and others were likely struggling to interpret the Supreme Court's guidance on issues with which they had little or no preparation or familiarity.

479. Indeed, it received renewed attention in *Zoloft Products Liability Litigation*, WL 3943916 (E.D.Pa, 2014).

480. *Brock v. Merrell Dow Pharm., Inc.*, 874 F.2d at 312 (a Bendectin plaintiff must proffer a statistically significant study before satisfying her burden of proof on causation); *Richardson v. Richardson-Merrell, Inc.*, 857 F.2d 823, 825, 831 n.59 (D.C. Cir. 1988), *cert. denied*, 493 U.S. 882 (1989) (noting that "epidemiological studies are of crucial significance"); and *Wade–Greaux v. Whitehall Laboratories, Inc.*, 874 F.Supp. 1441, (D.Vi.1994); see also *Daubert v. Merrell Dow Pharm. Inc.*, 43 F.3d 1311 (9th Cir.1995); and *Raynor v. Merrell Pharm. Inc.*, 104 F.3d 1371, 1375 (D.D.C.1997).

481. *Merck & Co., Inc. v. Garza*, 347 S.W.3d 256 (Tex. 2011). (Plaintiff must have two or more properly designed studies that show a doubling of the risk in question.)

482. Statistical studies utilize samples of a population to provide insights into a much-larger population. Sometimes samples may not represent the larger

population. Statisticians have devised methods to determine when the result from a sample might be mistaken because of small size. Statistical significance is a means of identifying the odds of a positive study—one showing an association between exposure and an adverse effect—being mistaken simply because of the statistics involved.

483. Oreskes, "Playing Dumb on Climate Change."
484. Steven N. Goodman and Richard Royall, "Evidence and Scientific Research," *American Journal of Public Health* 78.12 (1988): 1568–74; Charles Poole, "Beyond the Confidence Interval," *American Journal of Public Health* 77.2 (1987): 195–9; and Alexander M. Walker, "Reporting the Results of Epidemiologic Studies," *American Journal of Public Health* 76.5 (1986): 556–8. See also Carl F. Cranor, *Regulating Toxic Substances: A Philosophy of Science and the Law* (New York: Oxford University Press, 1993), 36–40 and 71–8, along with Michael D. Green, "Expert Witnesses and Sufficiency of Evidence in Toxic Substances Litigation: The Legacy of *Agent Orange* and Bendectin Litigation," *Northwestern University Law Review* 86.3 (1992): 691–2 (the chances of a false negative can easily be nearly 10 times the chances of a false positive).
485. Oreskes, "Playing Dumb on Climate Change."
486. See Hiroo Kato, "Cancer Mortality," in *Cancer in Atomic Bomb Survivors*, ed. Itsuzo Shigematsu and Abraham Kagan (Tokyo: Japan Scientific Societies Press, 1986), 53–74, quoted in Arthur K. Sullivan, "Classification, Pathogenesis, and Etiology of Neoplastic Diseases of the Hematopoietic System," in *Wintrobe's Clinical Hematology*, Vol. 1, 9th ed., ed. G. Richard Lee et al. (Philadelphia: Lea & Febiger, 1993), 1725, 1750.
487. Green, "Expert Witnesses" (one reviewer identified 71 epidemiologic studies that failed to satisfy statistical significance, but concluded that the "studies were consistent with a moderate or strong effect of the treatment under investigation" [at 685]). Jennie A. Freiman et al., "The Importance of Beta, the Type II Error and Sample Size in the Design and Interpretation of the Randomized Control Trial—Survey of 71 'Negative' Trials," *New England Journal of Medicine* 299.13 (1978): 690–4.
488. See Green, "Expert Witnesses," 686.
489. *Brock v. Merrell Dow Pharm., Inc.*, 874 F.2d 307.
490. IARC, *Special Issue: Combined Estrogen–Progestogen Contraceptives and Combined Estrogen–Progestogen Menopausal Therapy, IARC Monographs on the Evaluation of Carcinogenic Risks to Humans* 91 (2007), 54, available at http://monographs.iarc.fr/ENG/Monographs/vol91/mono91.pdf.
491. World Health Organization, "IARC Monographs Evaluate Consumption of Red Meat and Processed Meat," Press Release 240, October 26, 2015.
492. Ruth Etzel, Professor of Epidemiology at the University of Wisconsin's Joseph J. Zilber School of Public Health, pointed this out.

493. *Black v. Food Lion, Inc.,* 171 F.3d 308 (Fifth Circuit, 1999).

494. IARC administrators mention one such example out of hundreds of substances they have examined: "The complete sequence of steps in the metabolic activation of benzo[a]pyrene to mutagenic and carcinogenic diol epoxides has been demonstrated in experimental animals, in human tissues and cells, and in humans." (Cogliano, "Use of Mechanistic Data in IARC Evaluations," 106.)

495. *In re Agent Orange Product Liability Litigation,* 611F. Supp. 1223 (E.D.N.Y. 1985).

496. *Brock v. Merrell Dow Pharm., Inc.,* 874 F.2d 312 (a Bendectin plaintiff must proffer a statistically significant study before satisfying her burden of proof on causation).

497. Goldstein, "Toxic Torts: The Devil Is in the Dose," 556–7. "There is a commonality of biological function across [animal] species. All biological systems must obtain energy, build structure and release waste. The similarity in cellular and organ function is particularly strong . . . across mammals . . ."

498. IARC, "Preamble," section 2, *IARC Monographs on the Evaluation of Carcinogenic Risks to Humans* (rev. 2006).

499. IARC, "Preamble," section 8, *IARC Monographs on the Evaluation of Carcinogenic Risks to Humans* (rev. 2006).

500. Fabrice Larrazet et al., "Possible Bromocriptine-Induced Myocardial Infarction," *Annals of Internal Medicine* 118.3 (1993): 199–200.

501. IOM and NRC, *Dietary Supplements: A Framework for Evaluating Safety,* 134.

502. Ibid., 386–7, 399.

503. Henry Falk et al., "Hepatic Disease among Workers at a Vinyl Chloride Polymerization Plant," *Journal of the American Medical Association* 230.1 (1974): 59–63, at 59.

504. Clark W. Heath Jr. et al., "Characteristics of Cases of Angiosarcoma of the Liver among Vinyl Chloride Workers in the United States," in *Special Issue: Toxicity of Vinyl Chloride–Polyvinyl Chloride, Annals of the New York Academy of Sciences* 246 (January 1975): 231–36, at 231 (emphasis added).

505. IARC, "Preamble," *IARC Monographs on the Evaluation of Carcinogenic Risks to Humans,* 9. (These typically "arise from a suspicion, based on clinical experience, that the concurrence of two events—that is, a particular exposure and occurrence of a cancer [or other adverse effects] has happened rather more frequently than would be expected by chance.") They have provided "important information about the carcinogenicity of an agent . . . [and with other data] can add materially to the judgment that causation exists."

506. IARC, "4,4′-Methylenebis(2-Chlorobenzenamine)," in *Special Issue: Chemical Agents and Related Occupations, IARC Monographs on the Evaluation of Carcinogenic Risks to Humans* 100F (2012): 73–82, at 75 (explaining the carcinogenicity of MOCA as found in various experiments).

507. Ibid.

508. *Matrixx Initiatives, Inc. v. Siracusano,* 563 U.S. at 40–1.

509. *Allen v. Pennsylvania Engineering Corp. et al.,* 102 F.3d 194, at 198.

510. Cogliano et al, "Science and Practice," 2172. (The committees consider evidence that a substance causes cancer in humans and evidence that it causes cancer in animal studies to come to a presumptive conclusion, and this is then considered along with mechanistic and other kinds of evidence to "determine whether the default evaluation should be modified. . . . The final overall evaluation is a matter of scientific judgment, reflecting the *weight of the evidence derived from studies in humans, studies in experimental animals, and mechanistic and other relevant data*" [emphasis added].)

511. NRC, "Introduction," in *Review of Formaldehyde Assessment in the National Toxicology Program 12th Report on Carcinogens* (Washington, DC: National Academies Press, 2014), 4. ("Conclusions regarding carcinogenicity in humans or experimental animals are based on *scientific judgment,* with consideration given to *all relevant information.* Relevant information includes, but is not limited to, dose response, route of exposure, chemical structure, metabolism, pharmacokinetics, sensitive sub-populations, genetic effects, or other data relating to mechanism of action or factors that may be unique to a given substance" [emphasis added].)

512. Beron Roueche, "The Lemonade Mystery," *Saturday Evening Post,* May–June 1982, 59; Ronald C. Shank and Deborah C. Herron, "Methylation of Human Liver DNA after Probable Dimethylnitrosamine Poisoning," in *Nitrosamines and Human Cancer,* ed. Peter N. Magee (Cold Spring Harbor, NY: Cold Spring Harbor Laboratory Press, 1982), 153–9.

513. It points out that the plaintiff's argument in Allen was "at best weakly supported, if not contradicted, by the evidence on which they rely," whereas that was not true in *Milward.*

514. *Milward v. Acuity Specialty Products Group, Inc.,* 639 F.3d 11 (1st Cir. 2011), *rev'g* 664 F. Supp. 2d 137 (D. Mass. 2009), at 19.

515. David A. Eastmond (Chair, Environmental Toxicology Graduate Program, University of California, Riverside), personal communication; Austin Bradford Hill, "The Environment and Disease: Association or Causation?," *Proceedings of the Royal Society of Medicine* 58.5 (1965): 295–300, reprinted in *Evolution of Epidemiologic Ideas: Annotated Readings on Concepts and Methods,* ed. Sander Greenland (Chestnut Hill, MA: Epidemiology Resources, 1987), 15–20 (Hill implicitly endorses this form of reasoning by examples he cites).

516. Krimsky, "The Weight of Scientific Evidence in Policy and Law," S129.

517. Hill, "The Environment and Disease," 15–24. See also Douglas L. Weed, "Underdetermination and Incommensurability in Contemporary Epidemiology," *Kennedy Institute of Ethics Journal* 7.2 (1997): 107–24.

518. See, for example, Tom A. Hutchinson and David A. Lane, "Assessing Methods for Causality Assessment of Suspected Adverse Drug Reactions," *Journal of Clinical Epidemiology* 42.1 (1989): 5–16, at 12.

519. National Transportation Safety Board, *Aircraft Accident Report: In-Flight Breakup over the Atlantic Ocean; Trans World Airlines Flight 800, Boeing 747-131, N93119, near East Moriches, New York, July 17, 1996*, NTSB/AAR-00/03, DCA96MA070, PB2000-910403 (Washington, DC: National Transportation Safety Board, 2000), available at http://www.ntsb.gov/investigations/AccidentReports/Reports/AAR0003.pdf.

520. Carbone et al., "Modern Criteria," 5522. See also IOM and NRC, *Dietary Supplements*, 254. ("It is also not appropriate to develop a hierarchical approach to considering the different types of data—human data, animal data, *in vitro* data or information about related substances.... [S]uch an approach is not feasible because of limitations in the quality of the data and what different types of studies can reveal, but these limitations can be overcome with other types of data.")

521. IOM and NRC, *Dietary Supplements: A Framework for Evaluating Safety*, 255–6.

522. NRC, *Review of EPA's Integrated Risk Information System (IRIS) Process*, 80–104.

523. Cranor, *Toxic Torts*, 2nd ed., 295–306.

BIBLIOGRAPHY

Advisory Committee on Evidence Rules. "Proposed Amendment: Rule 702" (December 2011). Available at https://www.law.cornell.edu/rules/fre/rule 702.

Allen v. Pennsylvania Engineering Corp., 102 F.3d 194 (5th Cir. 1996).

American College of Obstetricians and Gynecologists Committee on Health Care for Underserved Women, American Society for Reproductive Medicine Practice Committee, with the assistance of the University of California at San Francisco (UCSF) Program on Reproductive Health and the Environment. "Committee Opinion: Exposure to Toxic Environmental Agents." Committee Opinion 575, October 2013.

American Law Institute. *Restatement (Second) of Torts.* (1965).

American Petroleum Institute. "Shanghai Studies: Internal Documents" (revealed in litigation), 1–163 (2003). [author has a copy]

Anway, Matthew D., Charles Leathers, and Michael K. Skinner. "Endocrine Disruptor Vinclozolin Induced Epigenetic Transgenerational Adult-Onset Disease." *Endocrinology* 147.12 (2006): 5515–23.

Applegate, John S. "Synthesizing TSCA and REACH: Practical Principles for Chemical Regulation Reform." *Ecology Law Quarterly* 35.4 (2008): 721–68.

Aristotle. *Nicomachean Ethics.* Translated by Terence Irwin. Indianapolis, IN: Hackett, 1985.

Bailar, J. C. Personal communication, 2004.

Bakke, Berit, Patricia A. Stewart, and Martha A. Waters. "Uses of and Exposure to Trichloroethylene in U.S. Industry: A Systematic Literature Review." *Journal of Occupational Environmental Hygiene* 4.5 (2007): 375–90.

Balibouse, Denis. "Teflon on Trial: Ohio Woman Wins $1.6mn Lawsuit Alleging DuPont Chemical Led to Cancer." *Reuters*, October 8, 2015. Available at https://www.rt.com/usa/318032-dupont-chemical-cancer-lawsuit/.

Barry, Vaughn, Andrea Winquist, and Kyle Steenland. "Perfluorooctanoic Acid (PFOA) Exposures and Incident Cancers among Adults Living near a Chemical Plant." *Environmental Health Perspectives* 121.11–12 (2013): 1313–8.

Bellinger, David, and Herbert L. Needleman. "The Neurotoxicity of Prenatal Exposure to Lead: Kinetics, Mechanisms and Expressions." In *Prenatal Exposure to Toxicants: Developmental Consequences*. Edited by Herbert L. Needleman and David Bellinger, 89–111. Johns Hopkins Series in Environmental Toxicology. Baltimore: Johns Hopkins University Press, 1994.

Berenson, Alex. "First Vioxx Suit: Entryway into a Legal Labyrinth?" *New York Times*, July 11, 2005. http://query.nytimes.com/gst/fullpage.html?res=9407E 7D81730F932A25754C0A9639C8B63.

Berger, Margaret A. "The Supreme Court's Trilogy on the Admissibility of Expert Testimony." In *Reference Manual on Scientific Evidence*. 2nd ed. Edited by Federal Judicial Center, 9–38. Washington, DC: Federal Judicial Center, 2000.

Berger, Margaret A. "The Admissibility of Expert Testimony." In *Reference Manual on Scientific Evidence*. 3rd ed. Edited by Federal Judicial Center, 11–36.Washington, DC: National Academies Press, 2011.

Betts, Kellyn S. "Perfluoroalkyl Acids: What Is the Evidence Telling Us?" *Environmental Health Perspectives* 115.5 (2007): A250–6. doi:10.1289/ehp.115-a250. PMC 1867999

Bienkowski, Brian. "Childhood Asthma, BPA Exposure Linked in New Study." *Environmental Health News*, March 1, 2013. Available at http://www.environmentalhealthnews.org/ehs/news/2013/asthma-and-bpa.

Bienkowski, Brian. "BPA Triggers Changes in Rats That May Lead to Breast Cancer." *Environmental Health News*, July 2, 2014. Available at http://www.environmentalhealthnews.org/ehs/news/2014/jul/bpa-mammary-glands.

Bienkowski, Brian. "BPA Exposure Linked to Changes in Stem Cells, Lower Sperm Production." *Environmental Health News*, January 22, 2015. Available at http://www.environmentalhealthnews.org/ehs/news/2015/jan/bpa-exposure-linked-to-changes-in-stem-cells-lower-sperm-production.

Bingham, E. Personal communication, 2004.

Birnbaum, Linda S., and Daniele F. Staskal. "Brominated Flame Retardants: Cause for Concern?" *Environmental Health Perspectives* 112.1 (2004): 9–17.

Black v. Food Lion, Inc., 171 F.3d 308 (5th Cir. 1999).

Blum v. Merrell Dow Pharmaceuticals, 33 Phila. Co. Rptr. 193–258 (1996).

Bouchard, Maryse F., Jonathan Chevrier, Kim G. Harley, Katherine Kogut, Michelle Vedar, Norma Calderon, Celina Trujillo, et al. "Prenatal Exposure to Organophosphate Pesticides and IQ in 7-Year-Old Children." *Environmental Health Perspectives* 119.8 (2011): 1189–95.

Braun, Joe M., Amy E. Kalkbrenner, Antonia M. Calafat, Kimberly Yolton, Xiaoyun Ye, Kim N. Dietrich, and Bruce P. Lanphear. "Impact of Early-Life Bisphenol A Exposure on Behavior and Executive Function in Children." *Pediatrics* 128.5 (2011): 873–82. Available at http://pediatrics.aappublications.org/content/early/2011/10/20/peds.2011-1335.

Brock v. Merrell Dow Pharmaceuticals, Inc., 884 F.2d 166 (5th Cir. 1989), modified, 884 F.2d 166 (5th Cir. 1989), cert. denied, 494 U.S. 1046 (1990).

Brown & Williamson Tobacco Company. "Smoking and Health Proposal." Doc. 680561778-1786, 1969, cited in David Michaels, *Doubt is their Product* (2012) p. 275.

California Environmental Protection Agency, Office of Environmental Health Hazard Assessment. "Guidance Criteria for Identifying Chemicals for Listing as 'Known to the State to Cause Cancer.'" Sacramento: California Environmental Protection Agency, Office of Environmental Health Hazard Assessment, 2001. Available at http://oehha.ca.gov/media/downloads/crnr/revcriteria.pdf.

Canfield, Richard L., Donna A. Kreher, Craig Cornwell, and Charles R. Henderson Jr. "Low-Level Lead Exposure, Executive Functioning, and Learning in Early Childhood." *Child Neuropsychology* 9.1 (2003): 35–53.

Cappiello, Dina. "Oil Industry Funds Study to Counter Cancer Claims." *Houston Chronicle*, April 29, 2005.

Carbone, Michele, George Klein, Jack Gruber, and May Wong. "Modern Criteria to Establish Human Cancer Etiology." *Cancer Research* 64.15 (2004): 5518–26.

Carson, Rachel. *Silent Spring*. New York: Houghton Mifflin, 1962.

Cecil, Kim M., Christopher J. Brubaker, Caleb M. Adler, Kim N. Dietrich, Mekibib Altaye, John C. Egelhoff, Stephanie Wessel, et al. "Decreased Brain Volume in Adults with Childhood Lead Exposure." *PLoS Medicine* 5.5 (2008): 741–50. Available at http://www.ncbi.nlm.nih.gov/pmc/articles/PMC2689675/pdf/pmed.0050112.pdf

Claxton, Larry D., Gisela de A. Umbuzeiro, and David M. DeMarini. "The *Salmonella* Mutagenicity Assay: The Stethoscope of Genetic Toxicology for the 21st Century." *Environmental Health Perspectives* 118.11 (2010): 1515–22.

Clermont, Kevin M., and Theodore Eisenberg. "Anti-plaintiff Bias in the Federal Appellate Courts." *Judicature* 84.3 (2000): 128–34.

Cogliano, Vincent James, Robert A. Baan, Kurt Straif, Yann Grosse, Béatrice Secretan, and Fatiha El Ghissassi. "Use of Mechanistic Data in IARC Evaluations." *Environmental and Molecular Mutagenesis* 49.2 (2008): 100–9.

Cogliano, Vincent James, Robert A. Baan, Kurt Straif, Yann Grosse, Béatrice Lauby-Secretan, Fatiha El Ghissassi, Véronique Bouvard, et al. "Preventable Exposures Associated with Human Cancers." *Journal of the National Cancer Institute* 103.24 (2011): 1827–39.

Cogliano, Vincent James, Robert A. Baan, Kurt Straif, Yann Grosse, Marie Béatrice Secretan, Fatiha El Ghissassi, and Paul Kleihues. "The Science and Practice of

Carcinogen Identification and Evaluation." *Environmental Health Perspectives* 112.13 (2004): 1269–74.

Cohn, Barbara A., Michele La Merrill, Nickilou Y. Krigbaum, Gregory Yeh, June-Soo Park, Lauren Zimmermann, and Piera M. Cirillo. "DDT Exposure in Utero and Breast Cancer." *Journal of Endocrinology & Metabolism* 100.8 (2015): 2865–72.

Cohn, Barbara A., Mary S. Wolff, Piera M. Cirillo, and Robert I. Sholtz. "DDT and Breast Cancer in Young Women: New Data on the Significance of Age at Exposure." *Environmental Health Perspectives* 115.10 (2007): 1406–14.

Collegium Ramazzini. "The Global Health Dimensions of Asbestos and Asbestos-Related Diseases." *European Journal of Oncology* 20.2 (2015): 121–6.

Cranor, Carl F. *Regulating Toxic Substances: A Philosophy of Science and the Law.* Environmental Ethics and Science Policy. New York: Oxford University Press, 1993.

Cranor, Carl F. "The Social Benefits of Expedited Risk Assessments." *Risk Analysis* 15.3 (1995): 353–8.

Cranor, Carl F. "Scientific Inferences in the Laboratory and the Law." In *Special Issue: Scientific Evidence and Public Policy. American Journal of Public Health* 95.S1 (2005): S121–8.

Cranor, Carl F. "A Framework for Assessing Scientific Arguments: Gaps, Relevance and Integrated Evidence." *Journal of Law and Policy* 15.1 (2007): 7–58.

Cranor, Carl F. *Legally Poisoned: How the Law Puts Us at Risk from Toxicants.* Cambridge, MA: Harvard University Press, 2011.

Cranor, Carl F. "*Milward v. Acuity Specialty Products*: Advances in General Causation Testimony in Toxic Tort Litigation." *Wake Forest Journal of Law & Policy* 3.1 (2013): 105–39.

Cranor, Carl F., and David A. Eastmond. "Scientific Ignorance and Reliable Patterns of Evidence in Toxic Tort Causation: Is There a Need for Liability Reform?" In *Special Issue: Causation in Law and Science. Law and Contemporary Problems* 64.4 (2001): 5–48.

Cranor, Carl F., John G. Fischer, and David A. Eastmond. "Judicial Boundary Drawing and the Need for Context-Sensitive Science in Toxic Torts after *Daubert v. Merrell Dow Pharmaceuticals, Inc.*" *Virginia Environmental Law Journal* 16 (1996): 1–77.

Daniels, Norman. "Health-Care Needs and Distributive Justice." *Philosophy and Public Affairs* 10.2 (1981): 146–79.

Daubert v. Merrell Dow Pharmaceuticals, Inc., 727 F.Supp. 570 (1989).

Daubert v. Merrell Dow Pharmaceuticals, Inc., 951 F.2d 1128 (9th Cir. 1991).

Daubert v. Merrell Dow Pharmaceuticals, Inc., 509 U.S. 579 (1993).

Denison, Richard A. *High Hopes, Low Marks: A Final Report Card on the High Production Volume Chemical Challenge.* Washington, DC: Environmental Defense, 2007.

Dennison, Richard A. "Historic Deal on TSCA Reform Reached, Setting Stage for a New Law after 40 Years of Waiting," Environmental Defense Fund (2016). Available at blogs.edf.org/health/2016/05/23/historic-deal-on-tsca-reform-reached-setting-stage-for-a-new-law-after-40-years-of-waiting/#more-5276.

Denison, Richard A. (Environmental Defense Fund). Email communication, January 11, 2014.

DES Action. "DES Timeline." Available at http://www.desaction.org/des-timeline/.

Dietert, Rodney R., and Michael S. Piepenbrink. "Perinatal Immunotoxicity: Why Adult Exposure Assessment Fails to Predict Risk." *Environmental Health Perspectives* 114.4 (2006): 477–83.

Dietert, Rodney R., and Judith T. Zelikoff. "Identifying Patterns of Immune-Related Disease: Use in Disease Prevention and Management." *World Journal of Pediatrics* 6.2 (2010): 111–8. doi: 10.1007/s12519-010-0026-1

DiMarini, David. Personal communication, 2012.

Dixon, Lloyd, and Brian Gill. *Changes in the Standards for Admitting Expert Evidence in Federal Civil Cases since the Daubert Decision.* Santa Monica, CA: RAND Institute for Civil Justice, 2001.

Donaldson v. Central Illinois Public Service, 767 N.E.2d 314 (2002).

Dufour-Rainfray, Diane, Patrick Vourc'h, Sébastien Tourlet, Denis Guilloteau, Sylvie Chalon, and Christian R. Andres. "Fetal Exposure to Teratogens: Evidence of Genes Involved in Autism." *Neuroscience & Biobehavioral Reviews* 35.5 (2011): 1254–65.

Eastmond, David A. Personal communication.

Ecobichon, Donald J. "Toxic Effects of Pesticides." In *Casarett and Doull's Toxicology: The Basic Science of Poisons.* 6th ed. Edited by Curtis D. Klaassen, 763–810. New York: McGraw-Hill, 2001.

Egilman, David S., and S. Rankin Bohme, eds. *Special Issue: Corporate Corruption of Science. International Journal of Occupational and Environmental Health* 11.4 (2005): 331–458.

Environmental Working Group. "Pollution in People: Cord Blood Contaminants in Minority Newborns." Environmental Working Group, 2009. Available at http://static.ewg.org/reports/2009/minority_cord_blood/2009-Minority-Cord-Blood-Report.pdf?_ga=1.260191565.19537483.1425936452.

"EPA, EDF, CMA Agree on Testing Program Targeting 2,800 Chemicals." *Environmental Health Newsletter* 37 (October 1998): 193.

Eriksson, Johan G., Tom Forsén, Jaakko Tuomilehto, Paul D. Winter, Clive Osmond, and David J. P. Barker. "Catch-Up Growth in Childhood and Death from Coronary Heart Disease: Longitudinal Study." *British Medical Journal* 318.7181 (1999): 427–31.

Eskenazi, Brenda, Jonathan Chevrier, Stephen A. Rauch, Katherine Kogut, Kim G. Harley, Caroline Johnson, Celina Trujillo, Andreas Sjödin, and Asa Bradman. "*In Utero* and Childhood Polybrominated Diphenyl Ether (PBDE) Exposures and Neurodevelopment in the CHAMACOS Study." *Environmental Health Perspectives* 121.2 (2013): 257–62. Available at http://ehp.niehs.nih.gov/wp-content/uploads/2012/11/ehp.1205597.pdf.

European Community, Registration, Evaluation, Authorisation, and Restriction of Chemicals (REACH), establishing a European Chemicals Agency, December 18, 2006, no. 1907/2006 (United Kingdom). For a more accessible generic guide, see http://www.reach-serv.com/index.php?option=com_content&task=view&id=121&Itemid=64.

Falk, Henry, John L. Creech Jr., Clark W. Heath Jr., Maurice N. Johnson, and Marcus M. Key. "Hepatic Disease among Workers at a Vinyl Chloride Polymerization Plant." *Journal of the American Medical Association* 230.1 (1974): 59–63.

Faustman, Elaine M., and Gilbert S. Omenn. "Risk Assessment." In *Casarett and Doull's Toxicology: The Basic Science of Poisons*. 6th ed. Edited by Curtis D. Klaassen, 83–104. New York: McGraw-Hill, 2001.

Fimrite, Peter. "Study: Chemicals, Pollutants Found in Newborns." *SFGate*, December 3, 2009. Available at http://www.sfgate.com/health/article/Study-Chemicals-pollutants-found-in-newborns-3207709.php.

Finley, Lucinda M. "Guarding the Gate to the Courthouse: How Trial Judges Are Using Their Evidentiary Screening Role to Remake Tort Causation Rules." *DePaul University Law Review* 49.2 (1999): 335–76.

Friedman, Lawrence M. *History of American Law*. 2d ed. New York: Touchstone, 1985.

Freiman, Jennie A., Thomas C. Chalmers, Harry Smith, and Roy R. Kuebler. "The Importance of Beta, the Type II Error and Sample Size in the Design and Interpretation of the Randomized Control Trial—Survey of 71 'Negative' Trials." *New England Journal of Medicine* 299.13 (1978): 690–4.

Frye v. U.S., 293 F.2d 1013 (D.C. Cir. 1923).

Furst, Arthur. "Yes, but Is It a Human Carcinogen?" *Journal of the American College of Toxicology* 9.1 (1990): 1–18.

Gale, Robert W., Walter L. Cranor, David A. Alvarez, James N. Huckins, Jimmie D. Petty, and Gary L. Robertson. "Semivolatile Organic Compounds in Residential Air along the Arizona-Mexico Border." *Environmental Science & Technology* 43.9 (2009): 3054–60.

Garner, Bryan A., ed. *Black's Law Dictionary*. 8th ed. St. Paul, MN: Thomson/West, 2004.

General Electric Company v. Joiner, 522 U.S. 136 (1997).

Gerona, Roy R., Tracey J. Woodruff, Carrie A. Dickenson, Janet Pan, Jackie M. Schwartz, Saunak Sen, Matthew W. Friesen, Victor Y. Fujimoto, and Patricia A. Hunt. "Bisphenol-A (BPA), BPA Glucuronide, and BPA Sulfate in Midgestation Umbilical Cord Serum in a Northern and Central California Population." *Environmental Science & Technology*. 47.21 (2013): 12477–85. Available at http://dx.doi.org/10.1021/es402764d.

Gilbert, Steven "Polybrominated Diphenyl Ethers (PBDEs)." Toxipedia: Connecting Science and People, 2014a (updated June 9). Available at http://www.toxipedia.org/pages/viewpage.action?pageId=296.

Gilbert, Steven. "Trichloroethylene." Toxipedia: Connecting Science and People, 2014b (updated June 9). Available at http://www.toxipedia.org/display/toxipedia/Trichloroethylene.

Gillette, Clayton P., and James E. Krier. "Risk, Courts, and Agencies." *University of Pennsylvania Law Review* 138.4 (1990): 1027–1109.

Goldman, Samuel M., Patricia J. Quinlan, G. Webster Ross, Connie Marras, Cheryl Meng, Grace S. Bhudhikanok, Kathleen Comyns, et al. "Solvent Exposures and Parkinson Disease Risk in Twins." *Annals of Neurology* 71.6 (2012): 776–84.

Goldstein, Bernard D. "Toxic Torts: The Devil Is in the Dose." *Journal of Law and Policy* 16.2 (2009): 551–87.

Goodman, Steven N., and Richard Royall. "Evidence and Scientific Research." *American Journal of Public Health* 78.12 (1988): 1568–74. Available at http://www.ncbi.nlm.nih.gov/pmc/articles/PMC1349737/pdf/amjph00251-0050.pdf.

Gottesman, Michael H. "From *Barefoot* to *Daubert* to *Joiner*: Triple Play or Double Error?" *Arizona Law Review* 40.3 (1998): 753–80.

Graham, Michael H. "The Expert Witness Predicament: Determining 'Reliable' under the Gatekeeping Test of *Daubert, Kumho*, and Proposed Amended Rule 702 of the Federal Rules of Evidence." *University of Miami Law Review* 54.2 (2000): 317–57.

Grandjean, Philippe, David Bellinger, Åke Bergman, Sylvaine Cordier, George Davey-Smith, Brenda Eskenazi, David Gee, et al. "The Faroes Statement: Human Health Effects of Developmental Exposure to Chemicals in Our Environment." *Basic & Clinical Pharmacology & Toxicology* 102.2 (2008): 73–5.

Grandjean, Philippe, Esben Budtz-Jørgensen, Dana B. Barr, Larry L. Needham, Pal Weihe, and Birger Heinzow. "Elimination Half-Lives of Polychlorinated Biphenyl Congeners in Children." *Environmental Science & Technology* 42.18 (2008): 6991–6.

Grandjean, Philippe, and Philip J. Landrigan. "Developmental Neurotoxicity of Industrial Chemicals." *The Lancet* 368.9553 (2006): 2167–78.

Greaves, Mel F., and Joe Wiemels. "Origins of Chromosome Translocations in Childhood Leukaemia." *Nature Reviews Cancer* 3.9 (2003): 639–49.

Green, Michael D. *Bendectin and Birth Defects: The Challenges of Mass Toxic Substances Litigation.* Philadelphia: University of Pennsylvania Press, 1996.

Green, Michael D. "The Road Less Well Traveled (and Seen): Contemporary Lawmaking in Products Liability." *DePaul Law Review* 49.2 (1999): 377–403.

Green, Michael D., D. Mical Freedman, and Leon Gordis. "Reference Guide on Epidemiology." In *Reference Manual on Scientific Evidence.* 2nd ed. Edited by Federal Judicial Center, 549–632. Washington, DC: Federal Judicial Center, 2000.

Grens, Kerry. "Effects of BPA Substitutes." In *Special Issue: Cancer's Grip. The Scientist* 30.4 (2016). Available at http://www.the-scientist.com//?articles.view/articleNo/45789/title/Effects-of-BPA-Substitutes/.

Griswold, Eliza. "How 'Silent Spring' Ignited the Environmental Movement." *New York Times Magazine*, September 21, 2012. Available at http://www.nytimes.com/2012/09/23/magazine/how-silent-spring-ignited-the-environmental-movement.html.

Gulf South Insulation v. Consumer Product Safety Commission, 701 F.2d 1137 (5th Cir. 1983).

Guth, Joseph H., Richard A. Denison, and Jennifer Sass. "Require Comprehensive Safety Data for All Chemicals." *New Solutions* 17.3 (2007): 233–58.

Haack, Susan. "An Epistemologist in the Bramble-Bush: At the Supreme Court with Mr. Joiner." *Journal of Health Politics, Policy and Law* 26.2 (1999): 217–48.

Harada, Masazumi. "Minamata Disease: Methylmercury Poisoning in Japan Caused by Environmental Pollution." *Critical Reviews in Toxicology* 25.1 (1995): 1–24.

Harr, Jonathan. *A Civil Action*. New York: Vintage, 1996.

Harremöes, David Gee, Malcolm MacGarvin, Andy Stirling, Jane Keys, Brian Wynne, and Sofia Guedes Vaz, eds. *Late Lessons from Early Warnings: The Precautionary Principle 1896–2000*. Environmental Issue Report 22. Copenhagen: European Environment Agency, 2001.

Harris v. CSX Transportation, Inc., 753 S.E.2d 275 (West Virginia Supreme Court, November 13, 2013).

Heath, Clark W., Jr., Henry Falk, and John L. Creech Jr. "Characteristics of Cases of Angiosarcoma of the Liver among Vinyl Chloride Workers in the United States." In *Special Issue: Toxicity of Vinyl Chloride–Polyvinyl Chloride. Annals of the New York Academy of Sciences* 246 (January 1975): 231–36.

Heath, David. "Meet the 'Rented White Coats' Who Defend Toxic Chemicals." Center for Public Integrity, February 8, 2016. Available at https://www.publicintegrity.org/2016/02/08/19223/meet-rented-white-coats-who-defend-toxic-chemicals.

Heindel, Jerrold J. "Animal Models for Probing the Developmental Basis of Disease and Dysfunction Paradigm." *Basic & Clinical Pharmacology & Toxicology* 102.2 (2008): 76–81.

Heinzow, Birger G. J. "Endocrine Disruptors in Human Breast Milk and the Health-Related Issues of Breastfeeding." In *Endocrine-Disrupting Chemicals in Food*. Edited by Ian Shaw, 322–55. Woodhead Publishing in Food Science, Technology, and Nutrition 170. Cambridge, UK: Woodhead, 2009.

Hilts, Philip J. *Protecting America's Health: The FDA, Business, and One Hundred Years of Regulation*. New York: Alfred A. Knopf, 2003.

Honda, Shun'ichi, Lars Hylander, and Mineshi Sakamoto. "Recent Advances in Evaluation of Health Effects on Mercury with Special Reference to Methylmercury—a Minireview." *Environmental Health and Preventive Medicine* 11.4 (2006): 171–6.

Honoré, Tony. "The Morality of Tort Law—Questions and Answers." In *Philosophical Foundations of Tort Law*. Edited by David G. Owen, 73–95. Oxford: Clarendon, 1995.

Hood, Ronald D. "Principles of Developmental Toxicology Revisited." In *Developmental and Reproductive Toxicology: A Practical Approach*. 2nd ed. Edited by Ronald D. Hood, 3–14. Boca Raton, FL: Taylor & Francis, 2006.

Hooper, Kim, and Thomas A. McDonald. "The PBDEs: An Emerging Environmental Challenge and Another Reason for Breast-Milk Monitoring Programs." *Environmental Health Perspectives* 108.5 (2000): 387–92.

Hoover, Sara M., Lauren Zeise, William S. Pease, Louise E. Lee, Mark P. Hennig, Laura B. Weiss, and Carl Cranor. "Improving the Regulation of Carcinogens by Expediting Cancer Potency Estimation." *Risk Analysis* 15.2 (1995): 267–80.

Huff, James. "Chemicals and Cancer in Humans: First Evidence in Experimental Animals." *Environmental Health Perspectives* 100 (April 1993): 201–10.

Huff, James, and David P. Rall. "Relevance to Humans of Carcinogenesis Results from Laboratory Animal Toxicology Studies." In *Maxcy-Rosenau-Last Public Health & Preventive Medicine*. 13th ed. Edited by John M. Last and Robert B. Wallace, 433–40, 453–57. Norwalk, CT: Appleton & Lange, 1992.

Hurtado v. Pharma Co., 6 Misc.3d 1015(A), 2005 WL 192351 (NY Sup. Ct. 2005).

In re: Agent Orange Product Liability Litigation, 611F. Supp. 1223 (E.D.N.Y. 1985).

In re Chantix (Varenicline) Products Liability, 889 F.Supp.2d 1272 (N.D.Ala.,2012).

In re Fosamax (Alendronate Sodium) Products Liability (not reported in F.Supp.2d, 2013 WL 1558690) (D.N.J.,2013).

Industrial Union Department, AFL-CIO v. Hodgson, 499 F. 2d 467 (1974).

International Agency for Research on Cancer. "Neutrons." In *Special Issue: Ionizing Radiation, Part 1: X- and Gamma (γ)-Radiation, and Neutrons. IARC Monographs on the Evaluation of Carcinogenic Risks to Humans* 75 (2000a): 363–448. Available at http://www-cie.iarc.fr/htdocs/monographs/ vol75/neutrons.html.

International Agency for Research on Cancer. "Etoposide." In *Special Issue: Some Antiviral Drugs, and Other Pharmaceutical Agents. IARC Monographs on the Evaluation of Carcinogenic Risks to Humans* 76 (2000b): 177–258. Available at http://www.inchem.org/documents/iarc/vol76/etoposide.html.

International Agency for Research on Cancer. "Preamble." *IARC Monographs on the Evaluation of Carcinogenic Risks to Humans*. Revised 2006. Available at http:// monographs.iarc.fr/ENG/Preamble/CurrentPreamble.pdf.

International Agency for Research on Cancer. *Special Issue: Combined Estrogen–Progestogen Contraceptives and Combined Estrogen–Progestogen MenopausalTherapy. IARC Monographs on the Evaluation of Carcinogenic Risks to Humans* 91 (2007). Available at http://monographs.iarc.fr/ENG/ Monographs/vol91/mono91.pdf.

International Agency for Research on Cancer. "Vinyl Bromide." In *Special Issue: 1,3-Butadiene, Ethylene Oxide and Vinyl Halides (Vinyl Fluoride, Vinyl Chloride and*

Vinyl Bromide). IARC Monographs on the Evaluation of Carcinogenic Risks to Humans 97 (2008a): 445–58. Available at http://monographs.iarc.fr/ENG/Monographs/vol97/mono97–9.pdf.

International Agency for Research on Cancer. "Vinyl Fluoride." In *Special Issue: 1,3-Butadiene, Ethylene Oxide and Vinyl Halides (Vinyl Fluoride, Vinyl Chloride and Vinyl Bromide). IARC Monographs on the Evaluation of Carcinogenic Risks to Humans* 97 (2008b): 459–72. Available at http://monographs.iarc.fr/ENG/Monographs/vol97/mono97–10.pdf.

International Agency for Research on Cancer. *Special Issue: Some Aromatic Amines, Organic Dyes, and Related Exposures." IARC Monographs on the Evaluation of Carcinogenic Risks to Humans* 99 (2010). Available at https://monographs.iarc.fr/ENG/Monographs/vol99/mono99.pdf.

International Agency for Research on Cancer. "Asbestos (Chrysotile, Amosite, Croccidolite, Tremolite, Actinolite, and Anthophyllite)." In *Special Issue: Arsenic, Metals, Fibres and Dusts. IARC Monographs on the Evaluation of Carcinogenic Risks to Humans* 100C (2012a): 219–309. Available at http://monographs.iarc.fr/ENG/Monographs/vol100C/index.php.

International Agency for Research on Cancer. "4,4'-Methylenebis(2-Chlorobenzenamine)." In *Special Issue: Chemical Agents and Related Occupations. IARC Monographs on the Evaluation of Carcinogenic Risks to Humans* 100F (2012b): 73–82. Available at http://monographs.iarc.fr/ENG/Monographs/vol100F/mono100F-9.pdf.

International Agency for Research on Cancer. "Formaldehyde." In *Special Issue: Chemical Agents and Related Occupations. IARC Monographs on the Evaluation of Carcinogenic Risks to Humans* 100F (2012c): 401–36. Available at http://monographs.iarc.fr/ENG/Monographs/vol100F/mono100F-430.pdf

International Agency for Research on Cancer. "Trichloroethylene." In *Special Issue: Trichloroethylene, Tetrachloroethylene, and Some Other Chlorinated Agents. IARC Monographs on the Evaluation of Carcinogenic Risks to Humans* 106 (2014): 35–218. Available at http://monographs.iarc.fr/ENG/Monographs/vol106/mono106-001.pdf.

Johns v. Bayer Corporation, 2013 WL 1498965 (S.D. Cal. Apr. 10, 2013).

Joiner v. General Electric Co., 78 F.3d 524 (11th Cir. 1996).

Julvez, Jordi, George D. Smith, Jean Golding, Susan Ring, Beate St. Pourcain, Juan Ramon Gonzalez, and Philippe Grandjean. "Prenatal Methylmercury Exposure and Genetic Predisposition to Cognitive Deficit at Age 8 Years." *Epidemiology* 24.5 (2013): 643–50.

Jurs, Andrew W., and Scott DeVito. "Et Tu, Plaintiffs? An Empirical Analysis of *Daubert*'s Effect on Plaintiffs, and Why Gatekeeping Standards Matter (a Lot)." *Arkansas Law Review* 66.4 (2013a): 975–1006.

Jurs, Andrew W., and Scott DeVito. "The Stricter Standard: An Empirical Assessment of *Daubert*'s Effect on Civil Defendants." *Catholic University Law Review* 62.3 (2013b): 675–731.

Kaati, Gunnar, Lars O. Bygren, and Soren Edvinsson. "Cardiovascular and Diabetes Mortality Determined by Nutrition during Parents' and Grandparents' Slow Growth Period." *European Journal of Human Genetics* 10.11 (2002): 682–8.

Kassirer, Jerome P., and Joe S. Cecil. "Inconsistency in Evidentiary Standards for Medical Testimony: Disorder in the Courts." *Journal of the American Medical Association* 288.11 (2002): 1382–87.

Kato, Hiroo. "Cancer Mortality." In *Cancer in Atomic Bomb Survivors*. Edited by Itsuzo Shigematsu and Abraham Kagan, 53–74. Gann Monograph on Cancer Research 32. Tokyo: Japan Scientific Societies Press, 1986. Quoted in Arthur K. Sullivan, "Classification, Pathogenesis, and Etiology of Neoplastic Diseases of the Hematopoietic System," in *Wintrobe's Clinical Hematology*, Vol. 1, 9th ed., edited by G. Richard Lee et al., 1725, 1750 (Philadelphia: Lea & Febiger, 1993).

Kaufman, Bruce. "Daubert Exclusions 'Haunt' Experts, but Need Not Be Career Ending Blows." *Bloomberg Occupational & Health Reporter* 46.14 (2016): 343–6.

Keeton, W. Page., ed. *Prosser and Keeton on the Law of Torts*. 5th ed. St. Paul, MN: West, 1992.

Kogevinas, Manolis, and Paolo Boffetta. "Letter to the Editor." *British Journal of Industrial Medicine* 48.8 (1991): 575–6.

Krimsky, Sheldon. "The Weight of Scientific Evidence in Policy and Law." *American Journal of Public Health* 95.S1 (2005): S129–36.

Kumho Tire Co. v. Carmichael, 526 U.S. 137 (1999).

Lan, Jiaqi, Man Hu, Ce Gao, Akram Alshawabkeh, and April Z. Gu. "Toxicity Assessment of 4-Methyl-1-Cyclohexanemethanol and Its Metabolites in Response to a Recent Chemical Spill in West Virginia, USA." *Environmental Science & Technology* 49.10 (2015): 6284–93. doi: 10.1021/acs.est.5b00371

Langston, J. William, and Phillip A. Ballard Jr. "Parkinson's Disease in a Chemist Working with 1-Methyl-4-Phenyl-1,2,5,6-Tetrahydropyridine." *New England Journal of Medicine* 309.5 (1983): 310.

Lanphear, Bruce P. "Origins and Evolution of Children's Environmental Health." In *Special Issue: Essays on the Future of Environmental Health Research: A Tribute to Kenneth Olden. Environmental Health Perspectives* 113 (August 2005): 1–3.

Larrazet, Fabrice, Christian Spaulding, Henri J. Lobreau, Simon Weber, and Francois Guerin. "Possible Bromocriptine-Induced Myocardial Infarction." *Annals of Internal Medicine* 118.3 (1993): 199–200. doi:10.7326/0003-4819-118-3-199302010-00008

Lerner, Sharon. "The Teflon Toxin: DuPont and the Chemistry of Deception." *The Intercept*, August, 11, 2015a. Available at https://theintercept.com/2015/08/11/dupont-chemistry-deception/.

Lerner, Sharon. "The Teflon Toxin: The Case against DuPont," *The Intercept*, August 17, 2015b. Available at https://theintercept.com/2015/08/17/teflon-toxin-case-against-dupont/.

Lerner, Sharon. "The Teflon Toxin: How DuPont Slipped Past the EPA." *The Intercept*, August 20, 2015c. Available at https://theintercept.com/2015/08/20/teflon-toxin-dupont-slipped-past-epa/.

Lerner, Sharon. "New Teflon Toxin Causes Cancer in Lab Animals." *The Intercept*, March 3, 2016. Available at https://theintercept.com/2016/03/03/new-teflon-toxin-causes-cancer-in-lab-animals/.

Lieb, David A. "Doe Run Settles Lead Liability Cases in Missouri." *Insurance Journal*, September 19, 2013. Available at http://www.insurancejournal.com/news/midwest/2013/09/19/305722.htm.

Lipton, Eric, and Rachel Abrams. "The Uphill Battle to Better Regulate Formaldehyde." *New York Times*, May 3, 2015. Available at http://www.nytimes.com/2015/05/04/business/energy-environment/the-uphill-battle-to-better-regulate-formaldehyde.html.

Loewen v. Wyeth, Inc. (not reported in F.Supp.2d, 2011) WL 6140889 (N.D.Ala., 2011).

Lombardi, Kristen. "Benzene and Worker Cancers: 'An American Tragedy.'" Center for Public Integrity, December 4, 2014. Available at http://www.publicintegrity.org/2014/12/04/16320/benzene-and-worker-cancers-american-tragedy.

Lyndon, Mary L. "The Toxicity of Low-Dose Chemical Exposures: A Status Report and a Proposal: Review of *Legally Poisoned: How the Law Puts Us at Risk from Toxicants.*" *Jurimetrics* 52.4 (2012): 457–500.

Maltoni, Cesare. "Predictive Value of Carcinogenesis Bioassays." In *Special Issue: Occupational Carcinogenesis. Annals of the New York Academy of Sciences* 271 (1976): 431–43.

Manikkam, Mohan, Carlos Guerrero-Bosagna, Rebecca Tracey, Md. M. Haque, and Michael K. Skinner. "Transgenerational Actions of Environmental Compounds on Reproductive Disease and Identification of Epigenetic Biomarkers of Ancestral Exposures." *PLoS ONE* 7.2 (2012): e31901. doi: 10.1371/journal.pone.0031901

Manikkam, Mohan, Rebecca Tracey, Carlos Guerrero-Bosagna, and Michael K. Skinner. "Dioxin (TCDD) Induces Epigenetic Transgenerational Inheritance of Adult Onset Disease and Sperm Epimutations." *PLoS ONE* 7.9 (2012): e46249.

Matrixx Initiatives, Inc. v. Siracusano, 563 U.S. 27 (2011).

Mayo Clinic Staff. "Diseases and Conditions: Infectious Diseases." Available at http://www.mayoclinic.org/diseases-conditions/infectious-diseases/basics/definition/con-20033534.

McCubbins, Matthew D., Roger G. Noll, and Barry R. Weingast. "Administrative Procedures as Instruments of Political Control." *Journal of Law, Economics, & Organization* 3.2 (1987): 243–77.

McHale, Cliona M., and Martyn T. Smith. "Prenatal Origin of Chromosomal Translocations in Acute Childhood Leukemia: Implications and Future Directions." *American Journal of Hematology* 75.4 (2004): 254–7.

McMillen, I. Caroline, and Jeffrey S. Robinson. "Developmental Origins of the Metabolic Syndrome: Prediction, Plasticity, and Programming." *Physiological Review* 85.2 (2005): 571–633.

Meeker, John D., Paula I. Johnson, David Camann, and Russ Hauser. "Polybrominated Diphenyl Ether (PBDE) Concentrations in House Dust Are Related to Hormone Levels in Men." *Science of the Total Environment* 407.10 (2009): 3425–9.

Michaels, David. *Doubt Is Their Product: How Industry's Assault on Science Threatens Your Health.* New York: Oxford University Press, 2012.

Michaels, David, and Celeste Monforton. "Manufacturing Uncertainty: Contested Science and the Protection of the Public's Health and Environment." *American Journal of Public Health* 95.S1 (2005): S39–S48.

Michaels, David, and Celeste Monforton. "How Litigation Shapes the Scientific Literature: Asbestos and Disease among Automobile Mechanics." *Journal of Law and Policy* 15.3 (2008): 1137–69.

Miller, Mark D., Melanie A. Marty, Amy Arcus, Joseph Brown, David Morry, and Martha Sandy. "Differences between Children and Adults: Implications for Risk Assessment at California EPA." *International Journal of Toxicology* 21.5 (2002): 403–18.

Milward v. Acuity Specialty Products Group, Inc., 639 F.3d 11 (First Circuit, 2011).

Milward v. Acuity Specialty Products Group, Inc., 664 F.Supp.2d 137, 140 (D.Mass.2009).

Mink v. University of Chicago, 460 F. Supp. 713 (1978).

Melman, Myron. Personal communication, 2012.

Michon, Kathleen. "Toxic Tort Litigation: Common Defenses." Nolo Law for All. Available at http://www.nolo.com/legal-encyclopedia/toxic-tort-litigation-common-defenses-32209.html.

Morris, Jim. "She Loved Making People Feel Great: Sandy Guest, 55, Hairdresser." Center for Public Integrity, June 29, 2015. Available at https://www.publicintegrity.org/2015/06/29/17533/she-loved-making-people-feel-great.

Morris, Jim. "Ford Spent $40 Million to Reshape Asbestos Science." Center for Public Integrity, February 16, 2016a. Available at http://www.publicintegrity.org/2016/02/16/19297/ford-spent-40-million-reshape-asbestos-science.

Morris, Jim. "About 'Science for Sale': The Danger of Tainted Science." Center for Public Integrity, February 18, 2016b. Available at http://www.publicintegrity.org/2016/02/08/19291/about-science-sale.

Nahar, Muna S., Chunyang Liao, Kurunthachalam Kannan, and Dana C. Dolinoy. "Fetal Liver Bisphenol A Concentrations and Biotransformation Gene Expression Reveal Variable Exposure and Altered Capacity for Metabolism in Humans." In *Special Issue: National Institute of Environmental Health Sciences Outstanding New Environmental Scientist Program. Journal of Biochemical and Molecular Toxicology* 27.2 (2013): 116–23. doi: 10.1002/jbt.21459

BIBLIOGRAPHY

National Research Council. *Risk Assessment in the Federal Government: Managing the Process.* Washington, DC: National Academy Press, 1983.

National Research Council. *Science and Judgment in Risk Assessment.* Washington, DC: National Academy Press, 1994.

National Research Council. *Review of Formaldehyde Assessment in the National Toxicology Program 12th Report on Carcinogens.* Washington, DC: National Academies Press, 2014.

National Research Council, Committee on Toxicity Testing and Assessment of Environmental Agents. *Toxicity Testing for Assessment of Environmental Agents: Interim Report.* Washington, DC: National Academies Press, 2006.

National Research Council, Steering Committee on Identification of Toxic and Potentially Toxic Chemicals for Consideration by the National Toxicology Program. *Toxicity Testing: Strategies to Determine Needs and Priorities.* Washington, DC: National Academy Press, 1984.

Navas-Acien, Ana, Eliseo Guallar, Ellen K. Silbergeld, and Stephen J. Rothenberg. "Lead Exposure and Cardiovascular Disease—a Systematic Review." *Environmental Health Perspectives* 115.3 (2007): 472–82.

Neiman, Max. *Defending Government: Why Big Government Works.* Upper Saddle River, NJ: Prentice Hall, 2000.

Nesson, Charles. "The Evidence or the Event? On Judicial Proof and the Acceptability of Verdicts." *Harvard Law Review* 98.7 (1985): 1357–92.

Nilsson, Eric, Ginger Larsen, Mohan Manikkam, Carlos Guerrero-Bosagna, Marina I. Savenkova, and Michael K. Skinner. "Environmentally Induced Epigenetic Transgenerational Inheritance of Ovarian Disease." *PLoS ONE* 7.5 (2012): e36129.

Oreskes, Naomi. "Playing Dumb on Climate Change." *New York Times,* January 3, 2015. Available at http://nyti.ms/1F0OIm6.

Perera, Frederica P., Wieslaw Jedrychowski, Virginia Rauh, and Robin M. Whyatt. "Molecular Epidemiologic Research on the Effects of Environmental Pollutants on the Fetus." *Environmental Health Perspectives* 107.S3 (1999): 451–60.

Pillard, Richard C., Laura R. Rosen, Heino Meyer-Bahlburg, James D. Weinrich, Judith F. Feldman, Rhoda Gruen, and Anke A. Ehrhardt. "Psychopathology and Social Functioning in Men Prenatally Exposed to Diethylstilbestrol (DES)." *Psychosomatic Medicine* 55.6 (1993): 485–91.

Poole, Charles. "Beyond the Confidence Interval." *American Journal of Public Health* 77.2 (1987): 195–9.

Rall, David P., Michael D. Hogan, James E. Huff, Bernard A. Schwetz, and Raymond W. Tennant. "Alternatives to Using Human Experience in Assessing Health Risks." *Annual Review of Public Health* 8 (1987): 355–85.

Rawls, John. *A Theory of Justice.* Rev. ed. Cambridge, MA: Belknap Press of Harvard University Press, 1999.

Rodgers, William H., Jr. *Environmental Law.* 2nd ed. St. Paul, MN: West, 1994.

Roe, Sam, and Patricia Callahan. "Distortion of Science Helped Industry Promote Flame Retardants, Downplay the Health Risks." *Chicago Sun Times,* May 9, 2012.

Ross, Julie A., Stella M. Davies, John D. Potter, and Leslie L. Robison. "Epidemiology of Childhood Leukemia, with a Focus on Infants." *Epidemiological Reviews* 16.2 (1994): 243–72.

Ruiz-Troche v. Pepsi Cola of Puerto Rico Bottling Company, 161 F. 3d 77 (1998).

Saks, Michael J. "Do We Really Know Anything about the Behavior of the Tort Litigation System—and Why Not?" *University of Pennsylvania Law Review* 140.4 (1992): 1147–1292.

Sass, Jennifer, and David Rosenberg. *The Delay Game: How the Chemical Industry Ducks Regulation of the Most Toxic Substances*. New York: Natural Resources Defense Council, 2011. Available at https://www.nrdc.org/sites/default/files/IrisDelayReport.pdf.

Savitz, David A., and Kurtis W. Andrews. "Risk of Myelogenous Leukaemia and Multiple Myeloma in Workers Exposed to Benzene." *Occupational and Environmental Medicine* 53.5 (1996): 357–8.

Schachtman, Nathan A. "WOE-fully Inadequate Methodology—an Ipse Dixit by Another Name." Available at http://schachtmanlaw.com/woe-ful-inadequate-methodology-an-ipse-dixit-by-another-name/.

Schardein, James L. *Chemically Induced Birth Defects*. 3rd ed., rev. and expanded. New York: Marcel Dekker, 2000.

Schardein, James L., and Orest T. Macina. *Human Developmental Toxicants: Aspects of Toxicology and Chemistry*. Boca Raton, FL: Taylor & Francis, 2007.

Schecter, Arnold, Olaf Päpke, Kuang Chi Tung, Jean Joseph, T. Robert Harris, and James Dahlgren. "Polybrominated Diphenyl Ether Flame Retardants in the U.S. Population: Current Levels, Temporal Trends, and Comparison with Dioxins, Dibenzofurans, and Polychlorinated Biphenyls." *Journal of Occupational & Environmental Medicine* 47.3 (2005): 199–211.

Schleifstein, Mark. "Dispersant Used in BP Spill Might Cause Damage to Human Lungs, Fish, Crab Gills, New Study Says." *Times-Picayune*, April 3, 2015. Available at http://www.nola.com/environment/index.ssf/2015/04/dispersant_used_in_bp_spill_mi.html.

Scierow, Linda-Jo. *The Toxic Substances Control Act (TSCA): A Summary of the Act and its Major Requirements*. Washington, DC: Congressional Research Service, Library of Congress, February 2, 2010.

Schierow, Linda-Jo. *The Toxic Substances Control Act (TSCA): Implementation and New Challenges*. CRS Report for Congress RL34118. Washington, DC: Congressional Research Service, Library of Congress, 2007.

Shulevitz, Judith. "Why Fathers Really Matter." Sunday Review, *New York Times*, September 8, 2012. Available at http://nyti.ms/QavdtZ.

Silbergeld, Ellen K., Daniele Mandrioli, and Carl F. Cranor. "Regulating Chemicals: Law, Science, and the Unbearable Burdens of Regulation." *Annual Review of Public Health* 36 (2015): 175–91.

Silbergeld, Ellen K., and Virginia M. Weaver. "Exposure to Metals: Are We Protecting the Workers?" *Occupational & Environmental Medicine* 64.3 (2007): 141–2.

Sindell v. Abbott Laboratories et al., 26 Cal.3d 588, 607 P.2d 924 (1980).

Singer, Natasha, and Duff Wilson. "Medical Editors Push for Ghostwriting Crackdown." *New York Times*, September 17, 2009. Available at http://www.nytimes.com/2009/09/18/business/18ghost.htm.

Skinner, Michael. Personal communication, September 20, 2014.

Skinner, Michael K., Mohan Manikkam, Rebecca Tracey, Carlos Guerrero-Bosagna, MuksitulHaque,andEricE.Nilsson."AncestralDichlorodiphenyltrichloroethane (DDT) Exposure Promotes Epigenetic Transgenerational Inheritance of Obesity." *BMC Medicine* 11 (2013): 228–50. doi: 10.1186/1741-7015-11-228. Available at http://www.ncbi.nlm.nih.gov/pmc/articles/PMC3853586/.

Smith, Martyn T. "Declaration of Martyn T. Smith" in *Milward v. Acuity Specialty Products*, March 9, 2009.

Steenland, Kyle, Liping Zhao, Andrea Winquist, and Christine Parks. "Ulcerative Colitis and Perfluorooctanoic Acid (PFOA) in a Highly Exposed Population of Community Residents and Workers in the Mid-Ohio Valley." *Environmental Health Perspectives* 121.8 (2013): 900–5. Available at http://dx.doi.org/10.1289/ehp.1206449.

Steinzor, Rena. "One Step Forward and Two Steps Back on Toxic Chemicals," Center for Progressive Reform. Available at http://www.progressivereform.org/CPRBlog.cfm?idBlog=DCC744AA-DE30-519C-874E812BFA8BE657 and at http://www.huffingtonpost.com/rena-steinzor/crossing-the-rubicon-on-t_b_10110578.html.

Swan, Shanna H., Katharina M. Main, Fan Liu, Sara L. Stewart, Robin L. Kruse, Antonia M. Calafat, Catherine S. Mao, et al. "Decrease in Anogenital Distance among Male Infants with Prenatal Phthalate Exposure." *Environmental Health Perspectives* 113.8 (2005): 1056–61.

Szabo, Liz. "Researchers Raise Concerns about BPA and Breast Cancer: Doctors Sound Alarm about Prenatal Health Hazards." *USA Today*, October 8, 2013. Available at http://www.usatoday.com/story/news/nation/2013/10/08/bpa-and-breast-cancer/2834461/.

Tomatis, Lorenzo, James Huff, Irva Hertz-Picciotto, Dale P. Sandler, John Bucher, Paolo Boffetta, Olav Axelson, et al. "Avoided and Avoidable Risks of Cancer." *Carcinogenesis* 18.1 (1997): 97–105.

Tracey, Rebecca, Mohan Manikkam, Carlos Guerrero-Bosagna, and Michael K. Skinner. "Hydrocarbons (Jet Fuel JP-8) Induce Epigenetic Transgenerational Inheritance of Obesity, Reproductive Disease and Sperm Epimutations." *Reproductive Toxicology* 36 (April 2013): 104–16.

Trasande, Leonardo, and Yinghua Liu. "Reducing the Staggering Costs of Environmental Disease in Children, Estimated at $76.6 Billion in 2008." *Health Affairs* 30.5 (2011): 863–70.

United States. *Federal Rules of Evidence*. Washington, DC: US Government Printing Office, 2000.

United States of America v. Philip Morris USA, Inc. et al., 449 F.Supp.2d 1 (D.D.C. 2006).

US Congress, Office of Technology Assessment. *Identifying and Regulating Carcinogens*. Washington, DC: US Government Printing Office, 1987.

US Consumer Product Safety Commission. "An Update on Formaldehyde." Publication 725, 2013 Revision 012013, 1–12. Washington, DC: US Consumer Product Safety Commission, 2013.

US Council on Environmental Quality. *Toxic Substances*. Washington, DC: US Government Printing Office, 1971.

US Department of Health and Human Services, Centers for Disease Control and Prevention. "Polychlorinated Dibenzo-p-Dioxins, Polychlorinated Dibenzofurans, and Coplanar and Mono-ortho-substituted Polychlorinated Biphenols." In *Third National Report on Human Exposure to Environmental Chemicals*. By US Department of Health and Human Services, Centers for Disease Control and Prevention, 135–200. Atlanta: US Department of Health and Human Services, Centers for Disease Control and Prevention, 2005. Available at http://www.jhsph.edu/research/centers-and-institutes/center-for-excellence-in-environmental-health-tracking/Third_Report.pdf.

US Department of Health and Human Services, Centers for Disease Control and Prevention, Agency for Toxic Substances and Disease Registry, Environmental Health and Medicine Education. "Trichloroethylene Toxicity: What Are the Physiological Effects of Trichloroethylene?" November 8, 2007. Available at http://www.atsdr.cdc.gov/csem/csem.asp?csem=15&po=10.

US Department of Health and Human Services, Public Health Service, National Toxicology Program. "Introduction." In *Thirteenth Report on Carcinogens*. Washington, DC: US Department of Health and Human Services, Public Health Service, National Toxicology Program, 2014. Available at http://ntp.niehs.nih.gov/ntp/roc/content/introduction_508.pdf.

US Department of Health and Human Services, Public Health Service, Office of the Surgeon General. "Cancer among Adults from Exposure to Secondhand Smoke." In *The Health Consequences of Involuntary Exposure to Tobacco Smoke: A Report of the Surgeon General*. Edited by Jonathan M. Samet, Leslie A. Norman, Caran Wilbanks, and Audrey Pinto, 421–506. Rockville, MD: US Department of Health and Human Services, Public Health Service, Office of the Surgeon General, 2006.

US Department of Health and Human Services, Task Force on Health Risk Assessment. *Determining Risks to Health: Federal Policy and Practice*. Dover, MA: Auburn House, 1986.

US EPA. "Assessing and Managing Chemicals under TSCA: Highlights of Key Provisions in the Frank R. Lautenberg Chemical Safety for the 21st Century Act." Available at https://www.epa.gov/assessing-and-managing-chemicals-under-tsca/highlights-key-provisions-frank-r-lautenberg-chemical.

US Environmental Protection Agency. "Appendix: The Toxic Substances Control Act; History and Implementation." Available at http://www.epa.gov/oppt/newchems/pubs/chem-pmn/appendix.pdf.

US Environmental Protection Agency. "EPA's New Chemicals Program under TSCA: The Basics." Available at http://www.chemalliance.org/topics/?subsec=27&id=689.

US Environmental Protection Agency. "High Production Volume (HPV) Challenge Program." US Environmental Protection Agency, 1999. Available at http://nepis. epa.gov/Exe/ZyNET.exe/7000052X.TXT?ZyActionD=ZyDocument&Client =EPA&Index=1995+Thru+1999&Docs=&Query=&Time=&EndTime= &SearchMethod=1&TocRestrict=n&Toc=&TocEntry=&QField=&QField Year=&QFieldMonth=&QFieldDay=&IntQFieldOp=0&ExtQFieldOp=0& XmlQuery=&File=D%3A%5Czyfiles%5CIndex%20Data%5C95thru99%5C Txt%5C00000019%5C7000052X.txt&User=ANONYMOUS&Password= anonymous&SortMethod=h%7C &MaximumDocuments=1&FuzzyDegree=0& ImageQuality=r75g8/r75g8/x150y150g16/i425&Display=p%7Cf&DefSeekPage =x&SearchBack=ZyActionL&Back=ZyActionS&BackDesc=Results%20page&M aximumPages=1&ZyEntry=1&SeekPage=x&ZyPURL.

US Environmental Protection Agency. "Trichloroethylene: Hazard Summary— Created in April 1992; Revised in January 2000." US Environmental Protection Agency, 2000. Available at https://www3.epa.gov/airtoxics/hlthef/tri-ethy.html.

US Environmental Protection Agency. "U.S. Federal Bans on Asbestos." US Environmental Protection Agency, 2016. Available at https://www.epa.gov/ asbestos/us-federal-bans-asbestos.

US Environmental Protection Agency, Office of Pesticide Programs. *General Principles for Performing Aggregate Exposure and Risk Assessments.* November 28, 2001. Available at https://www.epa.gov/sites/production/files/2015-07/ documents/aggregate.pdf.

US General Accounting Office. *Report to Congress: Toxic Substances Control Act; Legislative Changes Could Make the Act More Effective.* GAO/RCED-94-108. Washington, DC: US General Accounting Office, 1994.

US General Accounting Office. *Chemical Regulation: Options Exist to Improve EPA's Ability to Assess Health Risks and Manage Its Chemical Review Program.* GAO-05-458. Washington, DC: US General Accounting Office, 2005.

US Government Accountability Office. *Chemical Assessments: Low Productivity and New Interagency Review Process Limit the Usefulness and Credibility of EPA's Integrated Risk Information System.* GAO-08-440. Washington, DC: US Government Accountability Office, 2008.

US Institute of Medicine. *Identifying and Reducing Environmental Health Risks of Chemicals in Our Society: Workshop Summary.* Washington, DC: National Academies Press, 2014.

US Institute of Medicine and National Research Council, Committee on the Framework for Evaluating the Safety of Dietary Supplements. *Dietary Supplements: A Framework for Evaluating Safety.* Washington, DC: National Academy Press, 2005.

US National Institutes of Health, National Cancer Institute. "Diethystilbestrol (DES) and Cancer." Available at http://www.cancer.gov/cancertopics/causes-prevention/risk/hormones/des-fact-sheet.

U.S. Steel Corporation v. Milward, 132 S.Ct. 1002 (2012).

Vandenberg, Laura N., Theo Colborn, Tyrone B. Hayes, Jerrold J. Heindel, David R. Jacobs Jr., Duk-Hee Lee, Toshi Shioda, et al. "Hormones and Endocrine-Disrupting Chemicals: Low-Dose Effects and Nonmonotonic Dose Responses." *Endocrine Reviews* 33.3 (2012): 378–455.

vom Saal, Frederick F., Susan C. Nagel, Benjamin L. Coe, Brittany M. Angle, and Julia A. Taylor. "The Estrogenic Endocrine Disrupting Chemical Bisphenol A (BPA) and Obesity." In *Special Issue: Environment, Epigenetics and Reproduction. Molecular and Cellular Endocrinology* 354.1–2 (2012): 74–84.

Wade-Greaux v. Whitehall Lab., Inc., 874 F.Supp. 1441 (D.V.I.), aff'd, 46 F.3d 1120 (3d Cir. 1994).

Wade-Greaux v. Whitehall Lab., Inc., 46 F.3d 1120 (3d Cir. 1994).

Walker, Alexander M. "Reporting the Results of Epidemiologic Studies." *American Journal of Public Health* 76.5 (1986): 556–8.

Walter, Donna. "Missouri Lawyers of the Year Win $358M Toxic Tort Case." *Missouri Lawyer*, January 27, 2012. Available at http://molawyersmedia.com/2012/01/27/video-missouri-lawyers-of-the-year/.

Watson, James D., and Francis H. C. Crick. "Molecular Structure of Nucleic Acids: A Structure for Deoxyribose Nucleic Acid." *Nature* 171.4356 (1953): 737–8.

Wick, Peter, Antoine Malek, Pius Manser, Danielle Meili, Xenia Maeder-Althaus, Liliane Diener, Pierre-Andre Diener, Andreas Zisch, Harald F. Krug, and Ursula von Mandach. "Barrier Capacity of Human Placenta for Nanosized Materials." *Environmental Health Perspectives* 118.3 (2010): 432–6.

Wigle, Donald T., and Bruce P. Lanphear. "Human Health Risks from Low-Level Environmental Exposures: No Apparent Safety Thresholds." *PLoS Medicine* 2.12 (2005): e350.

Winter, Greg. "Jury Awards Soar as Lawsuits Decline on Defective Goods." *New York Times*, January 30, 2001. Available at http://www.nytimes.com/2001/01/30/business/30JURY.html?pagewanted=all.

Wong, Otto. "A Cohort Mortality Study and a Case-Control Study of Workers Potentially Exposed to Styrene in the Reinforced Plastics and Composites Industry." *British Journal of Industrial Medicine* 47.11 (1990): 753–62.

Woodruff, Tracey J., Lauren Zeise, Daniel A. Axelrad, Kathryn Z. Guyton, Sarah Janssen, Mark Miller, Gregory G. Miller, et al. "Meeting Report: Moving Upstream-Evaluating Adverse Upstream End Points for Improved Risk Assessment and Decision-Making." *Environmental Health Perspectives* 116.11 (2008): 1568–75.

Woodruff, Tracey J., Ami R. Zota, and Jackie M. Schwartz. "Environmental Chemicals in Pregnant Women in the United States: NHANES 2003–2004." *Environmental Health Perspectives* 119.6 (2011): 878–85.

World Health Organization. "IARC Monographs Evaluate Consumption of Red Meat and Processed Meat." Press Release 240, October 26, 2015.

Wright, Larry. *Practical Reasoning*. Edited by Robert J. Fogelin. San Diego, CA: Harcourt Brace Jovanovich, 1989.

INDEX